AF697574

THE SPREAD OF MEASLES IN FIJI AND THE PACIFIC

Spatial components in the transmission of epidemic waves through island communities

THE SPREAD OF MEASLES IN FIJI AND THE PACIFIC

Spatial components in the transmission of epidemic waves through island communities

ANDREW D. CLIFF
PETER HAGGETT

Department of Human Geography Publication HG/18
Research School of Pacific Studies
The Australian National University
Canberra

First published in Australia 1985
Printed in Australia for
The Australian National University

© The Australian National University 1985

This book is copyright. Apart from any fair dealing for the purpose of study, research, criticism, or review, as permitted under the Copyright Act, no part may be reproduced by any process without written permission. Inquiries should be made to the publisher.

National Library of Australia
Cataloguing-in-Publication entry

Cliff, Andrew D. (Andrew David), 1943-.

The spread of measles in Fiji and the Pacific.

Bibliography
ISBN 0 86784 733 6.

1. Measles - Fiji. 2. Measles - Pacific Area. I. Australian National University. Dept. of Human Geography. II. Haggett, Peter, 1933-. III. Title. (Series: Publication (Australian National University. Dept. of Human Geography); HG/18).

614.5'23'099

Department of Human Geography Publications are edited in the Department, in the Research School of Pacific Studies, The Australian National University, and are distributed by BIBLIOTECH, ANUTECH Pty Ltd, G.P.O. Box 4, Canberra, ACT 2601, Australia.

TABLE OF CONTENTS

LIST OF TABLES

LIST OF FIGURES

PREFACE

Our first studies of the geographical characteristics of epidemic spread were confined to the Northern mists of the sub-Arctic. We appreciate this opportunity provided by The Australian National University to explore this theme further in more congenial waters. Small islands provide, as Charles Darwin observed, remarkable field laboratories for many biological studies. This generalisation is nowhere truer than in the Pacific. The introduction of the measles virus into the populations of the Pacific in the second half of the 19th century provides a dramatic example of the demographic impact of disease and has been much studied. In this paper, we confine ourselves to the less-studied geographical aspects of that spread.

We are indebted to a number of people for their help and advice. In Australia, Peter Haggett had the privilege of working in the Department of Human Geography for a six month spell as a Visiting Fellow. He owes a special debt to The Australian National University in general, and to Gerard Ward and Harold Brookfield in particular, for many kindnesses and much advice over this period. The staff at the Menzies Library and the National Library in Canberra, and at the National Archives in Suva, proved unfailingly helpful. Dr Alan Tippett placed at our disposal his exceptional personal library at St Mark's in Canberra and gave advice based on his many years both as a Fijian scholar and a Methodist missionary in Fiji.

In Canberra, Pauline Falconer translated initial hieroglyphs into something a word processor could understand, and in Bristol, Margaret Reynolds carried on the battle with an ever-growing manuscript, this time made more difficult by two hands. Similarly with the drawings, Keith Mitchell and Lio Pancino in Australia, and Arthur Shelley and Simon Godden in England, converted rough sketches into figures. We are as grateful to them as to Bernard Devereux, who has designed a computer-based mapping system at Cambridge which we have been able to use.

Andrew Cliff
Peter Haggett

Chew Magna, England.
August 1984

CHAPTER 1

INTRODUCTION

PRELIMINARY REMARKS

Ever since Charles Darwin studied the finches of the Galapagos Islands in 1835, it has been recognised that oceanic islands can serve as large-scale laboratories for the investigation of biological processes.(1) Not long after Darwin completed his work, it became clear that remote islands, which offer a simpler site for study than the crowded continental mainland, can be used to enhance our understanding of the spread of disease. In the late 1840s Peter Panum, a Danish physician, made a study of the 1846 measles epidemic in the Faeroe Islands; this study has become one of the classic works of epidemiology (Panum, 1940), the discipline concerned with the patterns of disease in human populations. Today most advances in the study of diseases caused by viruses are made in laboratory conditions; for instance, the virus that causes measles was isolated in such a laboratory by John F. Enders and Thomas C. Peebles of the Harvard Medical School in 1954. Nevertheless, islands continue to play a significant role in elucidating how diseases spread under epidemic conditions.

Over the last decade, the authors have been part of an international team working on the modelling of the spatial spread of infectious diseases in general, and of measles and influenza in particular. The specifically geographical aspects of the work have been reported for measles in a series of papers with J.K. Ord of the Pennsylvania State University (see the account in Cliff et al., 1981). The work on the spread of influenza has been summarised in a study with epidemiologists, statisticians, environmental health officials and geographers published by the Sandoz Institute, Geneva (Selby, 1981).

The complexity of spatial spread processes in the continuously-distributed 'continental' populations such as those of northwest Europe has caused a shift towards the study of such processes in discontinuously-distributed 'island' communities. Significant work in isolated island populations in the Pacific region has been conducted by Brown et al. (1965, 1969), Gould et al. (1971) and Juptner and Quinnel (1965). This builds on the earlier work of Bartlett (1957) and F.L. Black (1966) which showed how community size and isolation could affect both the recurrence cycles of certain infectious diseases (Figure 1), as well as the shape and severity of individual epidemic waves. Figure 1A, based on Bartlett's work, indicates that the time gap between measles epidemics in communities is inversely related to their size. This implies that a critical population size (the Bartlett threshold) is required to sustain endemic infectious diseases. Populations above this threshold can be called Type I (Figure 1B). Just below this size threshold, epidemics will occur regularly but with well defined breaks in the disease sequence (Type II populations). Eventually, in still smaller populations, epidemics will occur only irregularly and be of variable magnitude (Type III populations). Black extended these ideas to islands and has shown that a unit in excess of 300,000 is needed to ensure endemicity for measles (Figure 1C). A mathematical basis for these changes had been provided by the theoretical work of N.T.J. Bailey at the World Health Organization (Bailey, 1975, 1981).

In this paper we first set out the rationale for working with island populations (Chapter 1). The main text is then divided into two chapters. In Chapter 2, Spatial Reconstruction, we look at the historical sequence in which measles arrived in the countries surrounding the Pacific and gradually spread from one island system to another. The islands of Fiji suffered particularly in this invasion process and the 1875 epidemic represents one of the greatest natural disasters in the history of the Pacific. This epidemic and several of its successors are examined.

Chapter 3, Spatial Analysis, is a quantitative account of the patterns formed by the measles epidemics which have affected the Pacific islands since the end of World War II. Time series methods are used to establish the geograpical and temporal components of spread. We look particularly at the relation of island systems to each other in this process. Here the critical questions relate to whether the Fijian outbreaks are to be regarded as independent events or whether they form part of some larger pan-Pacific system. We look for evidence of any convergence in behaviour over time between the various islands studied as the isolation of the area has been diminished by modern air and sea communications (Kissling, 1980; Taylor and Kissling, 1983).

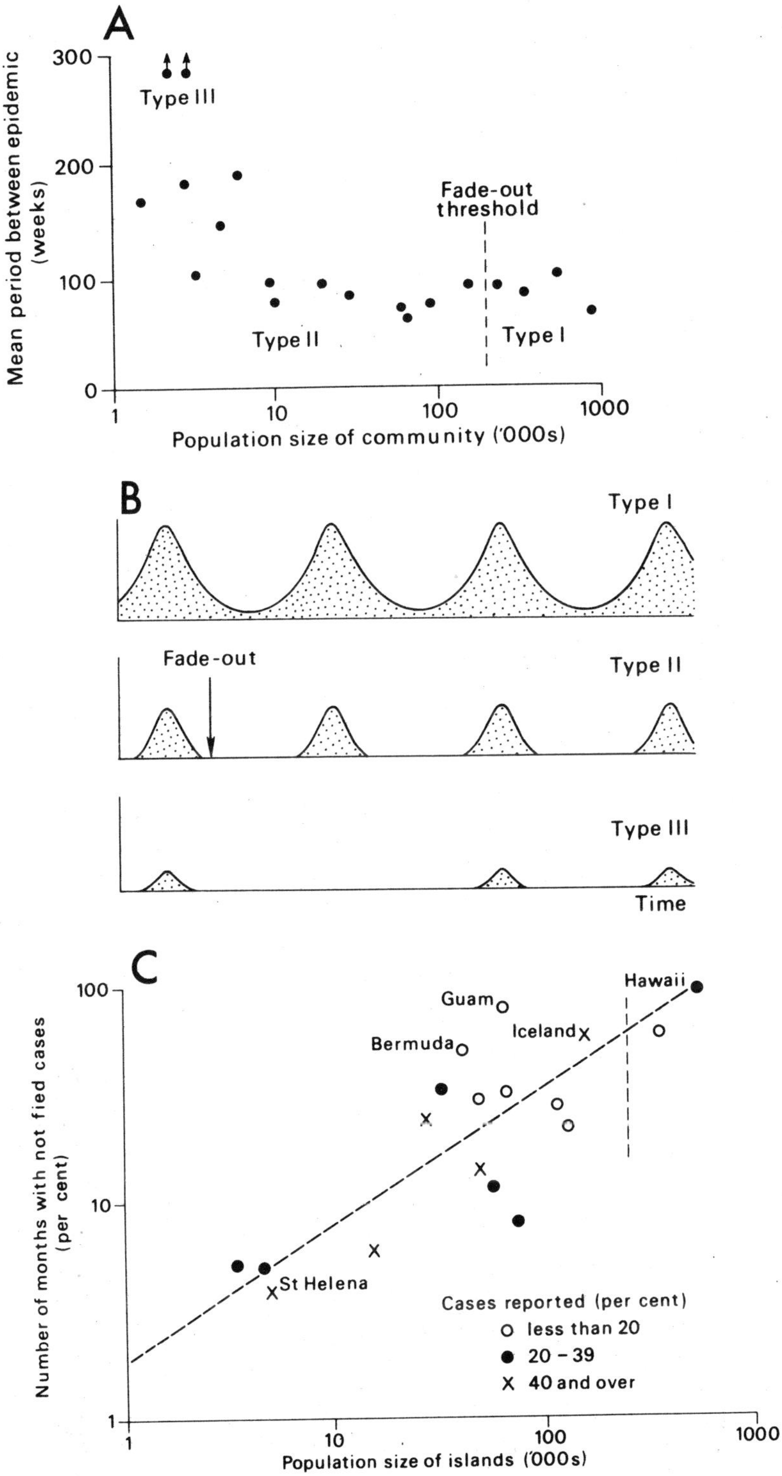

Figure 1: Epidemics and population size.

Although the study is retrospective and looks back over a century and a half of measles epidemics in the area, it is set in a context of rapid contemporary change. The campaign for measles elimination through vaccination which has proved so successful in the United States holds out the possibility of control and eventual elimination of the disease on a larger scale. We conclude our study on this optimistic note.

DESIGN OF THE STUDY

Geographers interested in contributing to an understanding of the spatial diffusion of epidemics can follow one of two main strategies. They can either reformulate and refine their general locational models to try to take account of the specific characteristics of the disease being diffused and the area through which it is spreading (Cliff et al., 1981), or they can isolate a specific real-world example of a spatial diffusion process and try to unravel the factors involved in the transmission process. In this paper, the second of the two approaches is followed. If such an approach is to produce generalisations about the spread process and not simply result in a narrowly conceived case study, careful attention must be paid to the selection of both the diffusion phenomenon to be studied and the geographical area in which its operation is to be analysed. It is to these issues which we now turn.

Islands as laboratories

A major difficulty in using continental areas within which to study epidemic spread is that it is effectively impossible to isolate geographical units which function as closed systems. As a result, disease leakage into and out of the area will be continuous. These swash and backwash effects will be difficult, if not impossible, to disentangle from the operation of the process within the area. By choosing islands for study, leakage will be reduced to a minimum and, importantly, these tend to occur at well-defined times when ships and aircraft bond the island units to continental areas. As a result, there is a greater chance of population flux (whether by migration, journey to work, tourism, or other passenger flows) being accurately recorded. Accurate estimation of the degree of population turbulence in terms of outflows and inflows plays an important part in any spatial epidemiological modelling.

For these reasons, much of the recent work undertaken by the authors has been focussed on island populations; the Icelandic study is continuing, while islands such as Gotland and Oland -- both off the Baltic coast of Sweden -- appear promising areas for further research.

The Pacific arena

The significance of island populations as a natural laboratory for geographical studies of diffusion leads easily to an interest in the Southwest Pacific. Here exist not only single islands isolated by vast tracts of ocean from their neighbours, but also island chains and islands closely linked to the Australian mainland.

The importance of the islands of the Southwest Pacific as research laboratories has been widely recognised. Thus H.E. Maude asked, in rhetorical mood, why we should bother with the detailed study of a region with - if we exclude New Guinea - 'a land area less than Cuba and a population less than Tehran' (Maude, 1968:xv), and answered his own question by using different islands as cameos of the colonial history of the area under different European powers. In a similar vein, the demographer, Norma McArthur, used different islands to compare and contrast features in the population history of the region.

Thus, in principle, the richness and diversity of island environments in this area should give an unparalleled opportunity for the development and testing of epidemiological models. Indeed, there are already some benchmark studies in the relevant literature (see the bibliographic review for Australia and New Zealand by Lancaster, 1964, 1973). However, whereas in the Scandinavian studies undertaken by the authors, epidemiological statistics were found to be exceptionally rich and to extend back in a partially usable form for some diseases into the late nineteenth century, inspection of the international records compiled by the World Health Organization suggests that data sets of this calibre are unlikely to be found for the Southwest Pacific. But useful comparative data do exist for the period since the Second World War. Even within this recent period, the different regulations and conventions of the administering governments, plus the varying levels of health provision, make records highly variable in reliability. While recent developments in categorical analysis make the statistical treatment of such variable data less difficult than a decade or so ago, major problems in data coverage and quality do remain and are addressed in Chapter 7.

Measles as a diffusion phenomenon

The way in which diseases endemic in the highly-populated continental areas of the world have been introduced by Europeans into the small island populations of the Pacific is one of the recurring themes in the history of the area. See for example, the definitive review by Norma McArthur in her Island Populations of the Pacific (1967). These diseases included influenza, leprosy, measles, mumps, smallpox, tuberculosis, typhoid, whooping cough and venereal disease, plus others which cannot be identified from the early historical records. From the long list of candidates, one disease - measles - is chosen here for special study.

The reasons for this choice have been argued at length elsewhere (Cliff et al., 1981:36-42) and relate principally to the geographical interest in diffusion waves which are replicable, stable over time and space, and observable. The specific advantages for measles are:

(a) The measles virus is one of the stable myxoviruses which, unlike influenza, does not appear to undergo major genetic changes. Measles outbreaks several decades apart can, on the basis of present virological knowledge, be assumed to be caused by the same viral agent. For the same reason, a measles attack may be assumed to give lifelong immunity.

(b) Measles has a simple and rather regular transmission mechanism which allows the virus to be passed from person to person. No intermediate host or vector is required. As the World Health Organization observes:

> The epidemiological behaviour of measles is undoubtedly simpler than that of any other disease. Its almost invariably direct transmission, the relatively fixed duration of infectivity, the lasting immunity which it generally confers, have made it possible to lay the foundations of a statistical theory of epidemics.(2)

It is, therefore, a disease whose spread can be modelled more readily than others.

Figure 2 shows the measles infection process as a chain structure. This gives a schematic model for measles contacts between an infective (i) and a susceptible (j). Open circles denote the onset of the infection. In the shortest chain (B), infective i makes contact on day 1 of his infectious period, and the susceptible j is 'latent' for as short a time as possible. The longest chain arises when i transmits on his last possible day of infection and j is latent for as long as possible (C). In the epidemiological literature, the average chain length (that is, the average time between the observation of symptoms in one case and the observation of symptoms in a second case directly infected from the first) is referred to as the 'serial interval' of the disease. For measles, this is about eleven to fourteen days.

(c) The disease is highly contagious with very high attack rates in an unvaccinated population. It generates, therefore, a very large number of cases over a short period of time to give a distinct epidemic wave. It occurs throughout the world without significant variation in relation to the ethnic or genetic background of the population infected or to the climatic environment in which they live.

(d) Measles has been a notifiable disease in a few countries since the 1880s and is currently recorded in more than sixty. The relative ease of clinical identification plus the high attack rates mean that the statistical reporting is less incomplete than for some other infectious diseases.

(e) Like smallpox, the measles virus is theoretically eradicable. Although the cost of global eradication is currently prohibitive, the campaign in the United States by the Center for Disease Control for the eradication of endemic measles has met with striking success (Hinman, 1982a,b). Study of the spatial structure of this particular disease is therefore likely to be usable in planning future eradication campaigns.

Thus, in summary, it is not chance which has led us to consider 'measles' and 'islands' for study, but a belief that their joint analysis gives better prospects for formulating and testing hypotheses, of leading to the development of models of the geographical diffusion of infectious disease, and finally of using such models in a way which promises to

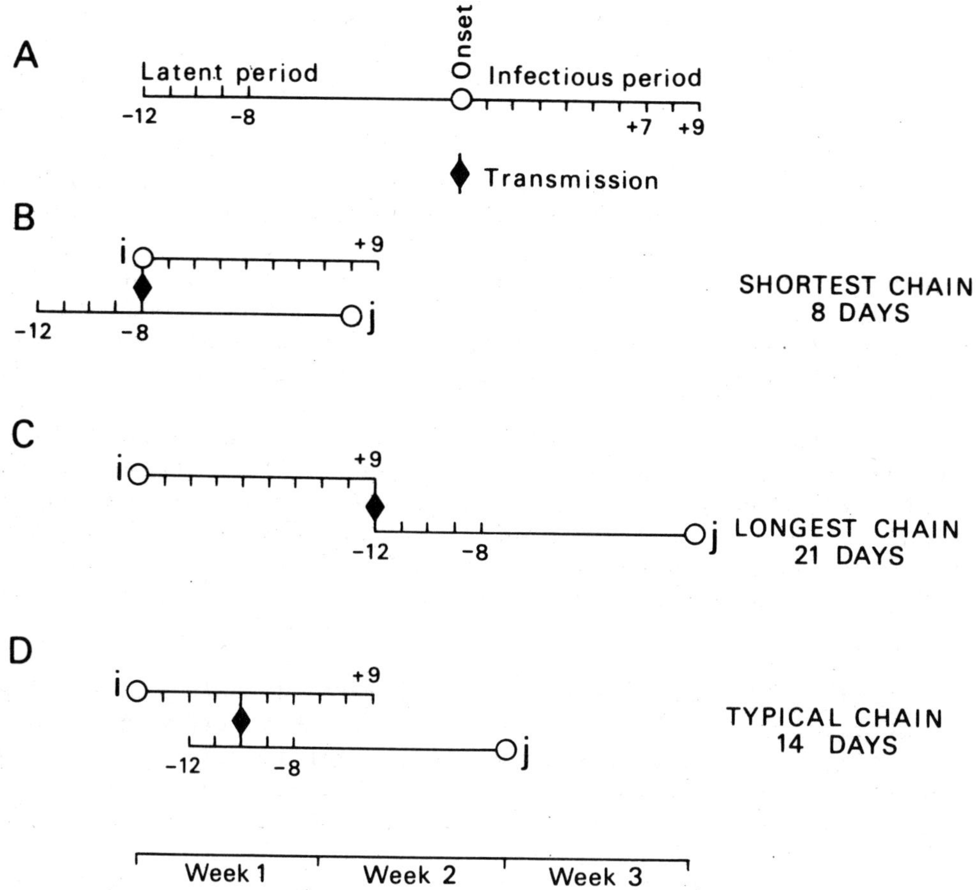

Figure 2: The infection process as a chain structure.

increase our understanding of the spread of a particular virus whose eradication as a public health problem is being actively sought.

NOTES

1. For a general account of island epidemics see Cliff and Haggett (1984).

2. World Health Organization, Epidemiological and Vital Statistics Report, Vol.5, p.332, August 1952.

CHAPTER 2

SPATIAL RECONSTRUCTION

INITIAL WAVES IN THE PACIFIC

As noted in the Introduction, a prime aim of this paper is to reconstruct the sequence of measles spread in the Pacific islands. This pattern is not made clear in the existing published literature, although such information as has appeared indicates that it may have arrived somewhat later than other infectious viral diseases. For example, Samoa experienced its first influenza epidemic in 1830 (introduced, ironically, by the missionary sailing ship, _Messenger of Peace_), its first whooping cough epidemic in 1848, and its first mumps epidemic in 1850. Conversely, measles did not reach the islands until 1893 (McArthur, 1967:102-09). Thus, in our reconstruction, attention is focussed on the nineteenth century and we look first at the situation at its start. Whether measles was introduced intermittently into the area before this date is a matter for conjecture; we can find no written records of such events (Ward and Hodge, 1967) and on theoretical grounds it seems highly unlikely.

The position in 1800

The spatial distribution, let alone the origin of measles, has never been mapped in detail. The earliest worldwide survey came from Hirsch at the University of Berlin who concluded in his great _Handbook of Geographical and Historical Pathology_ that the disease was 'in all probability widely diffused over Asiatic and European soil during the middle ages' (Hirsch, 1883, I:155). At that time it was absent from the Americas and Australasia, while the position in Africa south of the Sahara remains unresolved.

Portuguese settlement of eastern South America saw the establishment of measles in Brazil from the sixteenth century. In North America, measles appeared along the east coast in the seventeenth century. From there, Hirsch traces its westward spread following the settlement of the interior and the west coast. The most probable distribution of measles around the rim of the Pacific at the start of the nineteenth century is

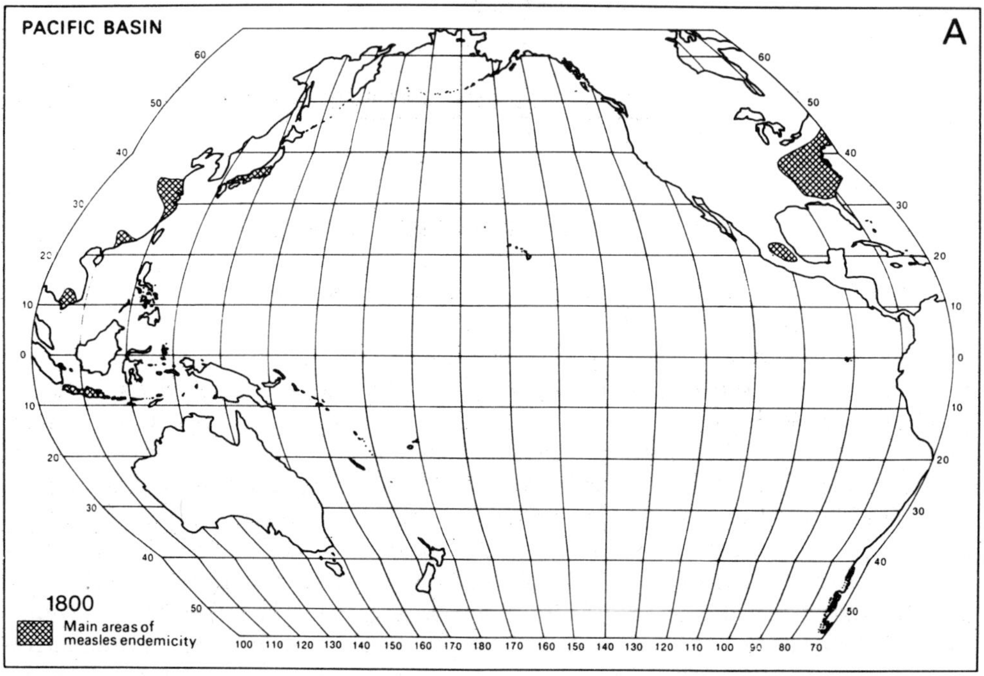

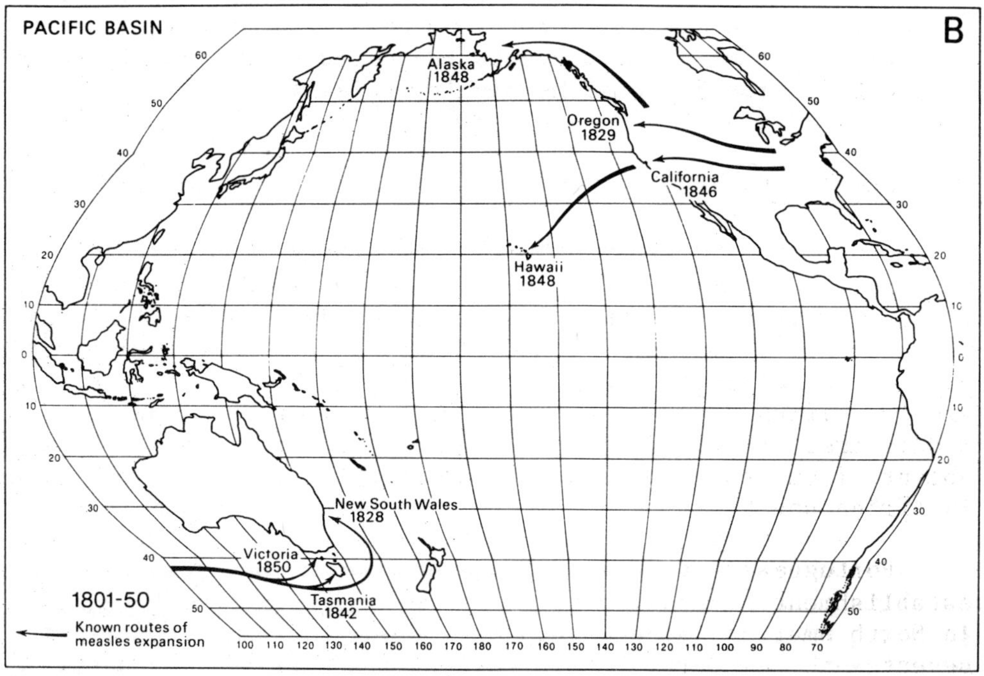

Figure 3: Generalised directions of measles spread in the Pacific Basin since 1800.

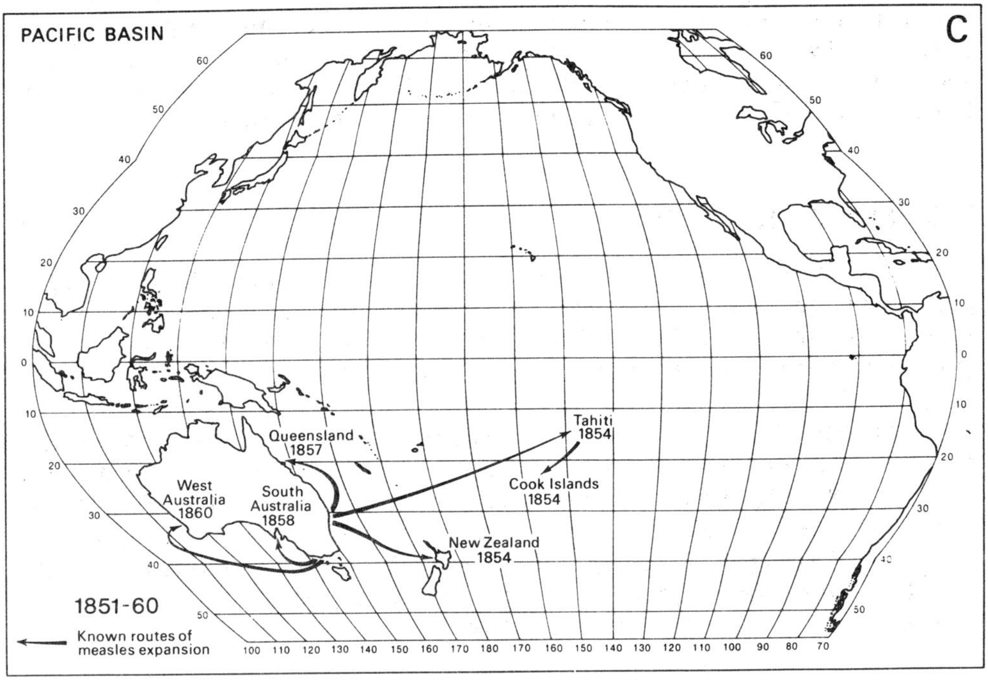

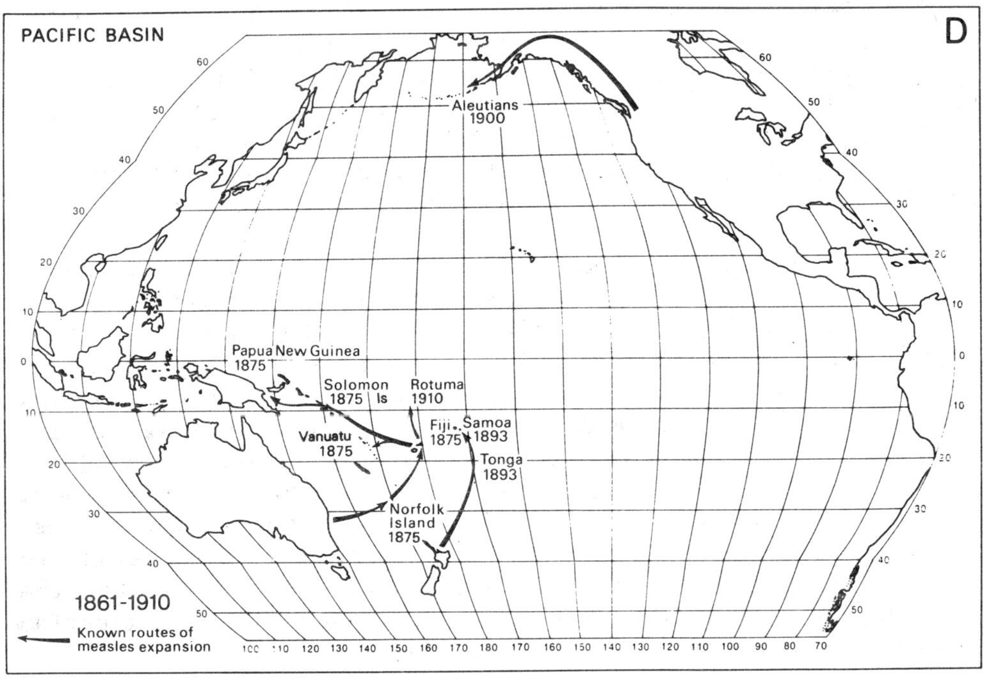

Figure 3: continued

shown in Figure 3A. It was endemic in the high-density population centres of South and East Asia and, by then, had most likely become established in central Mexico, and Peru and, less certainly, central Chile. It was unknown in the islands of the Pacific, Australia and New Zealand.

The nineteenth century

During the course of the nineteenth century this 'virgin soil' state was to be broken down and measles was introduced into most of the major island groups of the Pacific. The attack was to come from two major directions.

In the North Pacific the disease first appeared in Oregon in 1829 following the movements of the colonists westwards from the Mississippi Valley. It was recorded in California in 1846 and two years later had started an epidemic in the Hawaiian islands (Hirsch, 1883, I:158). Still further north, measles visited portions of the Alaskan peninsula in 1848 and Kodiak Island in 1875 (Wolfe, 1982).

In the South Pacific the main focus was Australia. So far as newspaper records allow, the arrival of measles on the Australian continent dates from 1828. Two years earlier the *Sydney Gazette* could proudly boast that 'measles has never been known in New South Wales or Victoria'(1), but in March 1828 the same paper reported that both measles and whooping cough had appeared in Sydney for the first time and that a quarantine of overseas ships was being observed.(2)

The subsequent spread of measles to the other Australian states has been traced in detail by J.H.L. Cumpston (1927). It appeared in Tasmania in 1842 and in Victoria in 1850. Within the next decade it had spread, apparently by secondary infection from the New South Wales-Victoria hearth, to New Zealand and to all the remaining states of Australia. The sequence runs: 1854 New Zealand, 1857 Queensland, 1858 South Australia, and 1860 Western Australia (see Figures 3B and 3C). There is sometimes doubt over small outbreaks which were confined to visiting ships; the dates in each case relate to major outbreaks which extended outside the port area into the rest of the state. The pattern of mortality in the Australian states from 1850 is shown in Figure 4.

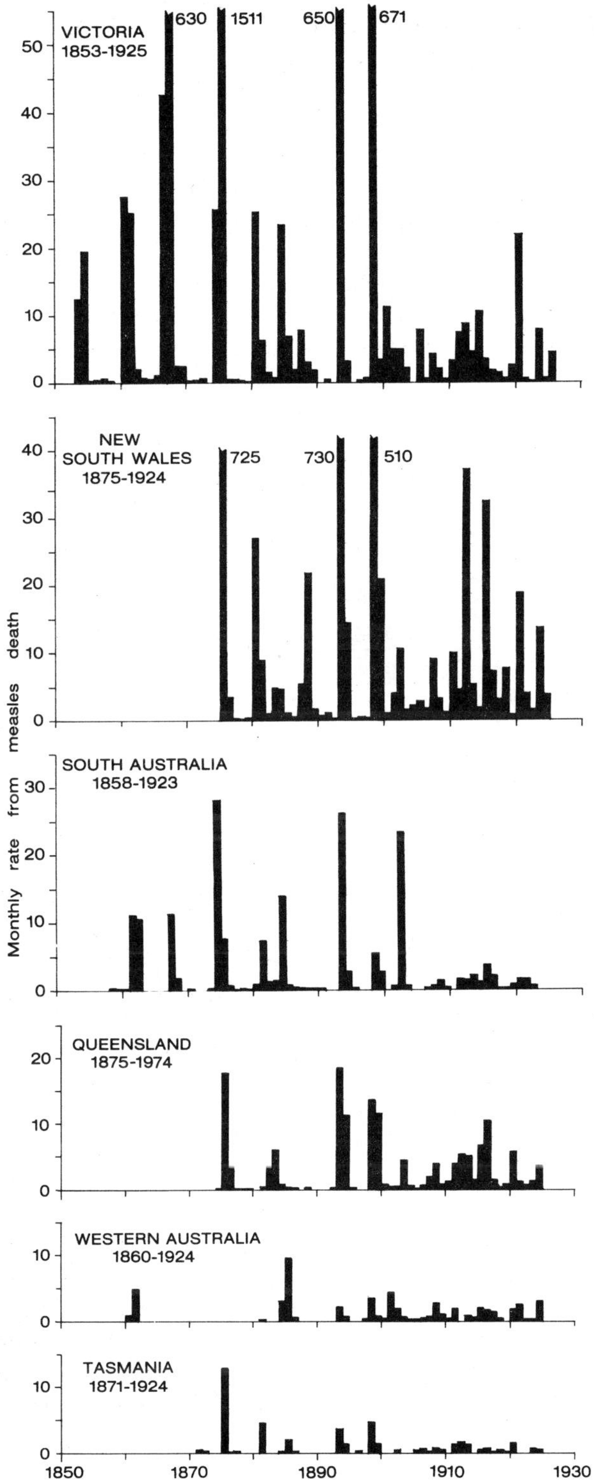

Figure 4: Death rate from measles in the Australian states, 1800-1924.

The spread of measles from Australia and New Zealand into the rest of the Southwest Pacific appears to have occurred in three distinct surges (Figure 3D). Much of the account which follows is based on the material reviewed by McArthur (1967).

Tahiti - Cook Islands, 1854. The first measles epidemic in French Polynesia started in April or May 1854 by an American vessel on her way from Newcastle, N.S.W. to San Francisco. In the same year the disease was introduced into the Cook Islands by a schooner from Tahiti. Mission correspondence includes reference to local outbreaks on the islands of Aitutaki and Mangaia in October of that year. Whether the infection was introduced into Rarotonga is less clear but, if so, this came in the last two or three weeks of the year. Although the evidence for mortality is ambiguous, there is no indication of widespread deaths and the only direct comment suggests the Cook Islands outbreak had been less severe than in Tahiti.

Fiji - Solomons - New Guinea, 1875. The introduction of measles into the Fijian group in January 1875 will be traced in detail in the next section. It is important to note that the ship which introduced measles to Fiji (HMS Dido) also infected Norfolk Island on the outward voyage and returned to Sydney via the Solomons; the first outbreak there may be attributable to that contact. In the same year measles was introduced into the southern Papuan coast of New Guinea by the London Missionary Society steamer Ellengowan.(3)

Tonga - Samoa, 1893. Although Tonga suffered a major epidemic soon after the Fiji disaster, probably about 1877 or 1878, this had very low mortality and is unlikely to have been measles. The first clear evidence of a measles outbreak on Tonga comes in 1893. The virus was thought to have been introduced from New Zealand (McArthur, 1967:76). The epidemic started in the southern island of Tongatapu and apparently spread through the whole island chain. Contemporary accounts (Thomson, 1894:286) suggest that, since the experience of Fiji eighteen years before was vivid in Tongan memories, they took some precautions against the after effects of the disease. Nevertheless, the death rate was very high and perhaps 1,000 people, some one twentieth of the Tongan population, succumbed to the disease. In 1893 Samoa also recorded its first measles epidemic (McArthur, 1967:109-11), but a link with Tonga has not been directly established.

The twentieth century

By 1900, measles had been introduced at least once into the major islands of the most-populated island groups of the Pacific and the disease was now endemic in two new 'bridgehead' areas - Australia and the west coast of North America. But there remained many smaller islands that were to remain free of contacts until this century. For example, most of the Aleutian Islands were not affected until 1900 and Rotuma, north of the main Fijian groups was not affected until 1911.

Whether small pockets of population which are virgin to measles remain in the Pacific today is the subject of current medical research. Examination of samples of sera for measles antibodies give an indication of whether an individual has been exposed to a measles virus attack. Thus, Willis and Warburton (1963) examined measles susceptibility on two Pacific atolls in the Papua New Guinea territory - Taku and Nukumanu. They concluded that since antibodies were absent in the majority of subjects of all ages, the virus had not been introduced into either atoll population within the lifetime of the present inhabitants. Where antibodies were found they were in subjects (mostly men over twenty) who had worked in major centres such as Bougainville Island or Rabaul where measles outbreaks had been known to occur.

Such seriological evidence is of course limited chronologically by the age of the oldest inhabitants; it also presumes that the migration history of the community is known. Given a sufficiently long interval between outbreaks (say, seventy years or more) it would be possible to have today a 'virgin soil' population all of whom were born since the last measles attack. This possibility was considered by Adels et al. (1963) in their study of measles antibodies from Ulithi and Ifalik atolls in the western Caroline Islands of Micronesia.

The existence of endemic reservoir areas for the measles virus in populations around the edge of the Pacific has clearly changed over time. If we accept Bartlett's estimate (Figure 1A) that a city with an unvaccinated population of about one quarter of a million can serve as a reservoir, then in 1800 we could only have found such concentrations in the north-west rim in the Japanese and Chinese populations. The dense rural population on the island of Java would also have served as such a base within the Indonesian archipelago.

TABLE 1: CITIES IN COUNTRIES AROUND THE PACIFIC BASIN WITH POPULATIONS ABOVE THE BARTLETT THRESHOLD[a]

Region 1 Pacific Islands	Region 2 Australia and New Zealand	Region 3 South and East Asia[b]	Region 4 North and South America
		A. UP TO 1850	
(None)	(None)	Nanjing Osaka Beijing Tokyo	(None)
		B. 1851 to 1900	
(None)	Melbourne(1873) Sydney(1877)	Kyoto(1860) Shanghai(1870) Hong Kong(1894)	Mexico City(1860) San Francisco (1885) Santiago(1894)
		C. 1901 to 1950	
Honolulu (1950)	Adelaide(1920) Brisbane(1924) Auckland(1936) Perth(1942)	Kobe(1904) Nagaya(1904) Manila(1907) Singapore(1909) Seoul(1909) Jakarta(1910) Surabaya(1915) Bangkok(1916) Taipei(1931) Saigon(1934) Bandung(1934) Vladivostok(1949) Kuala Lumpur(1950)	Los Angeles(1904) Portland(1905) Lima(1914) Seattle(1918) Vancouver(1932) Guatemala City (1944) Guayaquil(1948)

a Estimated at 250,000. Dates at which cities passed this threshold (given in brackets) is approximated by linear interpolation from population census. It should be noted that the estimation of city population size is notoriously imprecise and depends critically on local census definitions; these may vary from country to country and over time. An ideal epidemiological definition of a city would need to consist of the built-up city itself, plus an appropriate commuter zone based upon daily/weekly interactions. Sophisticated definitions of this kind are generally available only since 1950. The figures given above are based upon the legally-bounded area of the city and should therefore be used only to indicate broad geographical trends.

b Data for Chinese cities in the nineteenth century are sparse and the names given are an incomplete sample only.

As the nineteenth century progressed so the number of cities crossing the threshold increased. An estimate of the increased number of potential reservoir cities is given in Table 1, from six by 1850, to fourteen by 1900, and to nearly forty by 1950. The first Australian city (Melbourne) came of epidemiological age in 1873, the first city on the North American seaboard of the Pacific (San Francisco) in 1885. Within the Pacific itself, Honolulu remains the only city capable -- at any rate in theory -- of sustaining measles as an endemic disease. But as we note later (see Figure 16), the measles vaccination programme in Hawaii has proved so effective that Honolulu has now, in practice, only a very few imported cases in any one year.

INITIAL WAVES IN THE FIJI GROUP

The measles epidemic which engulfed the islands of the Fijian group(4) between January and June 1875 was one of the great tragic events of Pacific history (Squire, 1882). By the time the virus disappeared, one fifth (perhaps even one quarter) of the islands' population had perished.

The story has often been told and may well have gained something in the telling. The official report on the decrease of the native population(5) published eleven years after the end of the epidemic is concerned more with causes and cures than with a detailed reconstruction of spread. Likewise, much of the official correspondence nearer in time to the epidemic is concerned with avoiding blame rather than epidemiological description.(6) So in this section the account is restricted to two questions. First, what is the evidence and how accurate is it likely to be? Second, how far does it enable us to trace the geographical pattern of spread through the islands?

Source materials

A major epidemic involving a specific virus is an event in which we normally look primarily to medical evidence. In the first Fijian wave such evidence is almost entirely absent, because the arrival of measles just pre-dated the change to colonial status which was to bring a measure of medical organisation. At the height of the crisis, the situation was being coped with by just two medical officers(7), assisted on occasions by a ship's surgeon from a visiting vessel. How far the deaths which followed the introduction of measles were due to measles and its immediate sequelae and how much to associated diseases or malnutrition will never be known without ambiguity.

Even when William McGregor took up his duties as the first of Fiji's Chief Medical officers in June 1875 (at the very end of the epidemic) there were only four medical officers (Joyce, 1971:25) to serve 150,000 people scattered over 700,000 square miles on 300 islands, of which less than 100 were inhabited. Although some were outstanding and meticulous, some of the government doctors and the few private doctors in the colony were regarded by McGregor as being of poor quality. In 1887 one government doctor replied to the Chief Medical Officer's charge of insobriety in an unsteady hand:

> I was drunk both in Suva and here. I hate writing to you as I cannot help feeling I am writing to a 'Rabbit'. I await your instructions and will hand over my duties and my position to anyone but a mother-in-law.(8)

But positions were hard to fill and not all applicants for District Medical Officer posts held bona-fide medical qualifications. It was one of McGregor's many contributions to change this situation. The establishment was increased to eight by 1883 and a policy of recruiting young doctors from Scottish medical schools began to pay dividends. Fiji was to become a pace-setter in the provision of tropical medical services.

But all this was too late for the critical 1875 outbreak. For that we are dependent on correspondence, on newspaper accounts, and above all on mission papers. The first Wesleyan missionaries landed in eastern Fiji from Tonga in 1835 and the first Catholic mission was established in 1844. The conversion of the paramount chief of Lau in 1849 (and other chiefs thereafter) ushered in a period of remarkable expansion for the Wesleyan church. By 1875 the Wesleyans had an extensive chain of mission stations throughout the Fijian group. With its district organisation, its regular minutes and reports and its annual register of members, the records of the Wesleyan church were particularly suited to provide an indirect record of the mortality which accompanied the first great onslaught of the measles virus. Out of the sixteen circuits, eventually established, nine were in operation by

1875. Although the circuits have geographical names they may contain churches in widely-separated areas. For example, the records for the Yasawa Islands were included in the Bua records for many years. Although an inventory of documents has now been completed (Thornley, 1971), the researcher is faced with 109 shelf-feet of boxed records much of which contains no register or index system. Sampling from these papers in the National Archives in Suva suggests a more specific spatial picture might be built up for the 1875 outbreak but it would be a slow and incomplete process.

One of the main contributions of the mission records is to provide, from the list of adherents, a summed estimate of the loss of life in the first half of 1875. Whether due directly or indirectly to measles or not, the proportions revealed are awesome.

The spatial pattern of the initial wave

The first measles wave to strike the Fijian group was so disastrous in its impact and so rich in morbid detail that it forms a benchmark in Pacific history. It has been described in so many accounts(9) that only the bare outlines will be given here.

The opening phase. The first few links in the infectious chain can be plotted with some accuracy (Figure 5).

(i) The arrival of HMS *Dido* at the Fijian capital Levuka on the east coast of Ovalau Island on January 12th 1875 was the opening move (Figure 5A). The royal party on board, Cakobau and his two sons, were returning to Fiji after a state visit to New South Wales as guests of the governor, Sir Hercules Robinson. The Fijian chief had contracted measles while in Sydney and although the *Fiji Times* reported 'Cakobau looks anything but well after his trip'(10) he had long since ceased to be infectious. The vessel had left Sydney on 21st December but the two sons went down with measles during the twenty-two day voyage via Norfolk Island. On arrival at Levuka no yellow flag was flown and, although the disease was reported by the ship's surgeon, no attempt was made to stop either the welcoming group coming on board or the royal party disembarking. The status of the passengers, political sensitivity over cession, the lack of formal quarantine arrangements in Fiji, and a complete underestimate of the likely impact of measles in a virgin community all played some part in this oversight.(11)

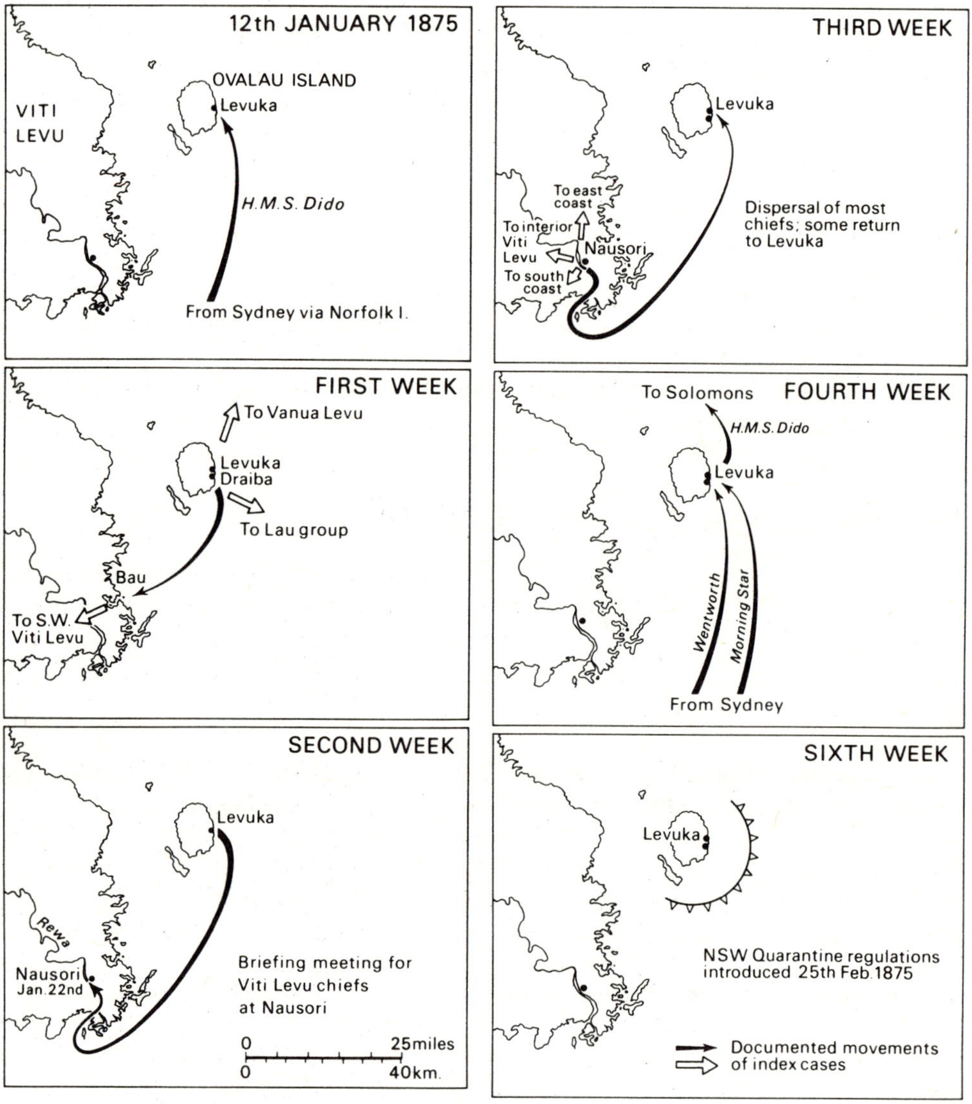

Figure 5: Elements in the spread of measles in the first few weeks of 1875 in Fiji (Wave I).

(ii) Over the course of the next ten days Cakobau entertained chiefs from Ovalau and the other islands at his homes at Draiba near Levuka and on the island of Bau (Figure 5B). An unusual number of high-ranking visitors came long distances both to welcome the senior chief home and to hear more about Fiji's new status as a British colony.

(iii) In the following week a major gathering of the chiefs of the hill tribes of Viti Levu was arranged at Navuso on the Rewa River (Figure 5C). About 800 appear to have gathered on January 22nd there to learn from the Administrator what cession meant. Some of the Ovalau chiefs and crew members of HMS Dido attended the meeting.

(iv) At the conclusion of the Navuso meeting, most hill chiefs went back to their homes but a small party of five of the most prominent (together with their groups) returned to Levuka to inspect the visiting warship (Figure 5D). By then Levuka was into its second generation of measles cases and the number of sick were multiplying alarmingly. All five chiefs were to die by the next month.

(v) The chiefs returned to their different parts of Viti Levu and HMS Dido sailed (in early February 1875) for Malekula in Vanuatu.

(vi) To make the epidemic bridgehead doubly secure, the Wentworth arrived at Levuka from Sydney on 26th January followed by the Western Star in early February (Figure 5E). Both carried active measles cases and, again, the infected passengers were allowed to land. It was to be February 25th before the quarantine laws of New South Wales were proclaimed in Fiji (Figure 5F).

It is important to note that we have direct medical evidence only of the two infected sons in link (i) and the passengers in (vi). That the virus was passed on during the other links (ii) to (v) is an inescapable inference from the news that began to come in from all parts of the island group. The unfortunate Dido returned workers from Fiji to the Solomons and Corney attributes the subsequent measles epidemic there and in the New Hebrides to this link (Corney, 1883-84:85).

While the speed of spread and intensity of impact is striking, it is hard to imagine a diffusion hierarchy more calculated to accelerate spread of the virus. At each point in the linkage pattern of Figure 5, we have an unusual number of people who have come long distances, who meet in close concourse, who then return to all parts of Fiji where they are met in their turn by local groups. The news about cession to Great Britain and the measles virus appear to have spread hand-in-hand downward through the layers of the social hierarchy.

Subsequent spread. The timing of the geographical spread of measles from then on is only partly known. Ovalau and Bau were clearly infected in early January and the returning chiefs could have spread the virus into most districts by late January or early February. Reports from mid-February confirm the presence of measles in all provinces and 'by the early or middle part of March disastrous news came in from all quarters' (Corney, 1883-84:80). The peak incidence of the disease was reached in the original centres (Ovalau and Bau) toward the end of March, and in most other places by early April. The eastward Lau group was last affected but measles appear to have spread, albeit at a slower rate, into all the major islands including Ono-i-Lau, 390 km from Levuka.

The end of the epidemic showed a similar spatial pattern. By the middle of April, good news began to appear in the Fijian press. A correspondent from Rewa wrote on April 20th that:

> The measles are on the decrease and with the continuance of the present fine weather the natives will soon all be well.(12)

By early May it had died out in Ovalau and the more accessible parts of Viti Levu; by early June it had disappeared from the whole group, so that by the time the colony's first Chief Medical officer arrived, the epidemic was over.

The disappearance of measles from the Lau group is confirmed by correspondence between McGregor and the Colonial Secretary. Writing on September 7th 1875, McGregor draws attention to the 842 deaths since the visit of the *Barracouta* in the early part of the year, but by August 'with the exception of Ono and Vatea [Vatoa] the measles have entirely disappeared and the general health of the natives is good'.(13) He later confirms in an interview with a Mr Young from the island of Ono, that

> The epidemic is now over and the general health is

> pretty much the same as in the other windward islands. He does not think there was a single case of measles there when he left [August 1875] and does not think it necessary to send down a medical officer as there is nothing special now requiring his presence, and as the epidemic has run itself out.(14)

It is not clear from the correspondence precisely when the last case occurred, but it seems unlikely that the outbreak could have prolonged itself beyond the middle of the year on any scale.

The demographic impact. The full impact of measles on the Fijian population will never be known. The 'unrecorded' pre-1881 census, taken in 1879, showed a count of 108,924 Fijians plus an estimated 3,000 working on European plantations. The official estimate of the population of the Fijian group at the start of 1875 was 150,000 and the final estimate of deaths was 'not less than 40,000' (Corney, 1883-84:84). This would give a death rate of around 27 per cent.

The origins of these official estimates are obscure and recent research has tended to question them. McArthur, after an extended review of the evidence, suggests that a total pre-epidemic population nearer to 135,000 (and certainly not over 140,000) is more likely. If we applied the same number of deaths as in the official estimates then the death rate rises to 30 per cent; but if we retain the same rate (27 per cent) and apply it to the smaller population, then the total deaths fall to 36,000. Precise estimates for deaths in the first half of 1875 are not available. As we might expect, the rate fluctuates from community to community but is generally lower than in the official rate. It appears from these figures that the death rate of 1:5 rather than 1:4 would be a more realistic assessment. If we combine this with McArthur's lower population estimate then the loss of life might be as low as 27,000. The real figure probably lies somewhere between this figure and the official estimate of 40,000, not The Times figure of 50,000.(15)

The best estimates of deaths at the local level come from the class registers and records of the Methodist Church (Tippett, 1953). An example is given in Table 2. This emphasises the widely varying attack rates between one island and another, and between one village and another. Detailed reconstruction of the geography of deaths will depend on the careful analysis of documents such as that in Appendix 1. Clearly, whatever the exact number, the measles epidemic of 1875 was a tragedy of the first order.

TABLE 2: SPATIAL VARIATION IN THE ESTIMATED DEATH RATE FROM MEASLES[a] FOR MEMBERS OF METHODIST CHURCHES IN LAU (THE WINDWARD ISLANDS), 1875[b]

Circuit level	Section level	DR	n			Village level[c]	DR	n
	Totoya	137	[75]					
	Komo	192	[20]					
	Matuku	229	[162]			7 villages		
	Lakeba	258	[210]	--	MIN.	Yadrana	127	[20]
					MAX.	Nukunuku	459	[17]
Lakeba 279 per 1000 [1119 deaths]	Moala	259	[205]					
						4 villages		
	Fulaga	342	[107]	--	MIN.	Ogea	12	[1]
					MAX.	Naividamu	493	[36]
	Kabara	363	[107]					
	Moce	383	[59]					
	Namuka	435	[54]					
	Oneata	755	[120]					

a Death rate per thousand. Number of deaths on which the rate is based follows in square brackets.

b Records from the Lakeba Circuit Minute Book in the Methodist Missionary Archives, Suva [Lau/A/1], given in Tippett (1974:31-2).

c Details at village level for only two of the ten sections.

LATER WAVE SEQUENCES IN THE FIJI GROUP

In this section, the historical sequence of measles waves recorded in the Fijian group is summarised. It is important to note that the record is a partial one and that, especially in the earlier decades, one cannot be sure that small outbreaks which were brief in duration and affected only isolated islands in the group were recorded.

TABLE 3: CHARACTERISTICS OF FIJI'S MAIN MEASLES EPIDEMICS, 1875 TO PRESENT

Wave	Years (with months where known)	Measures of measles incidence: Recorded deaths	Hospital admissions	Reported cases
I	1875 (1)-(7)	c.40,000[a]	(b)	(b)
II	1903	c. 2,000[a]	(b)	(b)
III	1910-14	344	400	(b)
IV	1921	0	195	(b)
V	1927	1	165	(b)
VI	1936-37	1	215	6,700
VII	1946 (1) - 47 (2)	2	(c)	4,856
VIII	1957 (2)-(11)	35	(c)	7,059
IX	1963 (8) - 64 (12)	1	32	7,375
X	1967 (4) - 68 (9)	2	1	4,517
XI	1971 (2) - 72 (9)	(c)	(c)	7,152
XII	1973 (12) - 76 (3)	(c)	(c)	3,046
XIII	1976 (11) - 78 (1)	(c)	(c)	2,477
XIV[d]	1978 (12) - 81 (2)	(c)	(c)	2,588

a Estimates only. See discussion in text.

b Not recorded.

c Recorded but not published in Annual Medical Reports for Fiji.

d A fifteenth measles wave which peaked in 1982 occurred too late for it to to be included in the study.

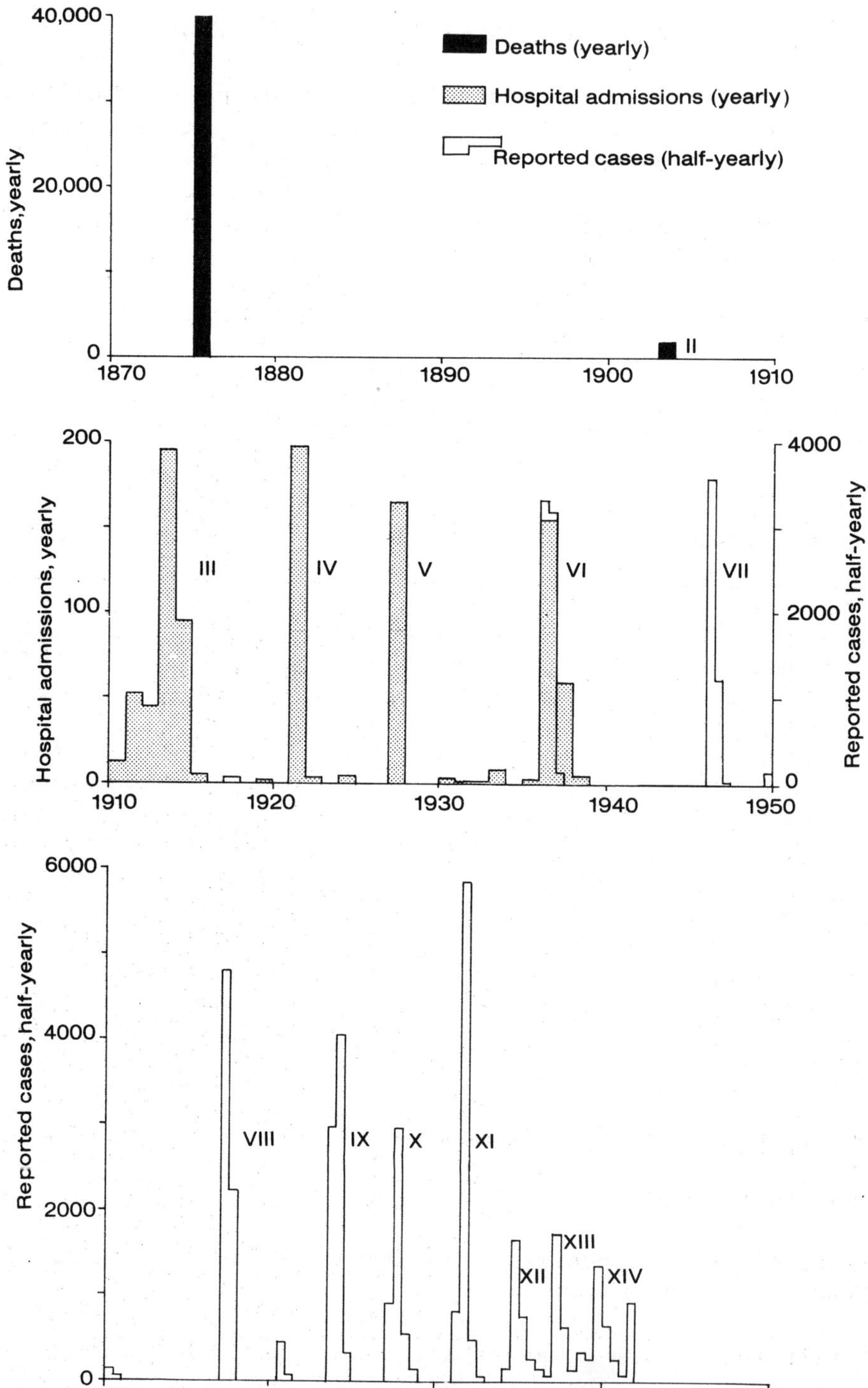

Figure 6: Sequence of measles waves in Fiji from 1875 to present.

By using the combined records from several sources, the broad picture of measles activity in Fiji can be traced (Table 3). It must be emphasised that all three measures -- deaths, hospital admissions, and reported cases -- must be treated with very great reserve. In each case, the figures are likely to be considerable underestimates. It is, however, one of the virtues of measles that it produces such an abundance of cases in its epidemic phases that these clearly stand out from the episodes when the virus is entirely absent or only sporadic cases are occurring.

Figure 6 shows in a composite diagram a sequence of fourteen distinct waves from 1875 to the early 1980s. The evidence for the first two waves is based on annual mortality estimates for deaths from measles and its sequelae. Waves II to VI are identifiable from figures for hospital admissions for measles given in the *Annual Medical Reports*, while from Wave VI to the present, the admission figures, when available, are supplemented by the monthly totals for notified cases as reported originally to the League of Nations Health Section and subsequently to the World Health Organization.

The periods between epidemics are not necessarily devoid of measles cases. Sporadic cases are likely, particularly at seaports from imported cases, but there is a distinct difference in magnitude and intensity between the major waves, each of which involve more than one thousand (and up to more than 100,000 cases in 1875) and the small-scale and spatially limited outbreaks which sometimes occur between them.

Wave II: the evidence of measles mortality

A notice given by the Colonial Secretary under the Public Health ordinance in September 1893 gives a vivid picture of the attitude to measles in the years following the initial wave:

> The Governor invites earnest public attention to the fact that Measles are prevalent at all the principal ports of New Zealand and Australia. In the latter place the disease is reported by medical authority to be of a severe type, and the same authority expresses the opinion that Measles will spread over the whole of the Colonies and extend to the Islands of the Pacific. As a matter of fact the disease has already reached Tonga and Samoa...Having regard to

> the frequency of communication between Sydney and New Caledonia the probabilities are that Noumea must shortly be included among the Infected Ports if it should not already be so included. Thus as regards the disease named the Colony may be regarded as 'in the state of siege'; and most stringent precautions are necessary.(16)

The notice goes on, in apocalyptic terms to remind readers what happened twenty years before and to confidently invite 'the sympathetic and active cooperation of all classes of the public in contending with the dangers which are now threatening'. In due course measles cases did land in Suva but were immediately quarantined; no major epidemic developed. Thus, although there were to be sporadic outbreaks from imported cases (such as that in 1880 when 17 cases developed on the Waimanu estates from a Sydney visitor) they were small, short-lived and highly localised. It was nearly three decades after 1875 before the next islands-wide outbreak.

The evidence for the size of this 1903 outbreak is largely retrospective. Writing in May 1913, Fiji's Chief Medical Officer, looking back over the changing impact of measles, noted that the natives, when they do contract the disease, do not suffer as they did in the former epidemics of 1875 and 1903. For 1903 he states that

> the epidemic was so universal and so serious that probably now the only natives left to have it are those who have been born since that date.(17)

A similar retrospective review was conducted by Lynch's successor in May 1922. But this refers to the disease being kept out of Fiji by quarantine from 1874 to 1903 when 'a very serious epidemic then occurred with over 2000 deaths'.(18) Since no medical officer's report can be traced for the two years in the Fiji legislative council papers and there is no reference in the Blue Books for that period, there is no direct evidence on the timing or extent of the disease. The lack of press comment at the time on the 1903 outbreak is surprising. It seems likely that the many outbreaks which had occurred over the intervening twenty-eight years had all been so small in scale and so localised to the port areas that even this larger wave caused little public concern.

Waves III to VI: the evidence of hospital admissions

Source materials. The rapid fall in measles mortality this century means that morbidity rather than mortality data become critical and here the accuracy of the data depends on medical priorities and practices. The first sixty years of Fiji's colonial medical services were guided by only five Chief Medical Officers: W. McGregor (1875-86), B. Glanville Corney (1886-1908), G.W.A. Lynch (1909-18), A. Montague (1919-28) and A.B.H. Pearce (1930-37). Each laid emphasis on slightly different priorities of medical care and each chose to record, retain and publish health statistics in a slightly different way.

The Annual Medical Reports which were published regularly since 1909 provide the main source for epidemiological information. Lynch, who had himself served as a District Medical Officer for twenty years included the district reports as part of his annual report when he took over from Corney in 1908. This practice was continued until 1930 and gives valuable spatial information on the presence of localised epidemics which affected only some districts within the island group. After 1930, the reports become more streamlined with more emphasis on hospital activities, but from 1936 this is partly compensated by Pearce's inclusion of tables for infectious diseases. Tables continue to be included up to the present day, but their format and level of detail are rather inconsistent, so that it is not possible to assemble an unbroken series.

For much of the period covered by the next four measles waves (1911 to 1938) the most consistent set of data for measles incidence comes from hospital admissions. The structure which was built up to provide medical hospital services in Fiji was an intricate one. Figure 7 shows the multi-tier structure which had been constructed by the end of World War II. At the top of the hierarchy was the Colonial War Memorial Hospital at Suva, with its specialist facilities and associated Medical School. It admitted more than twice the number of cases of the largest of the three district hospitals at Lautoka on the western side of Viti Levu. The other two provincial hospitals, at the two islands of Vanua Levu (Labasa) and Ovalau (Levuka), were smaller but well equipped.

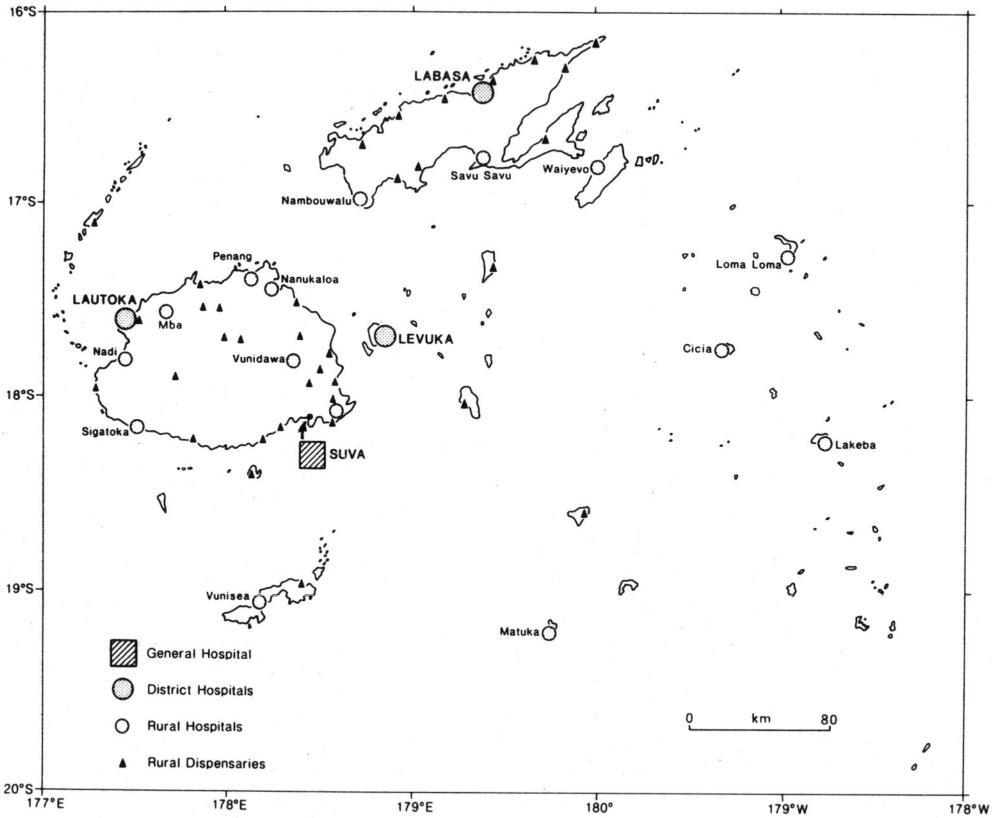

Figure 7: Provision of hospital facilities in Fiji by the end of 1945.

Below the district hospitals on the third tier of the hierarchy were seventeen rural hospitals. Seven of these were on Viti Levu, two on Vanua Levu, and the remainder widely spread through the smaller islands. On the lowest tier of the medical care system were a further thirty-six rural dispensaries widely spread through the main islands. It is interesting to note that, in the eastern Lau group, the rural hospital tends to be the most frequent unit, possibly as a special arrangement to cope with the very scattered pattern of population in the archipelago. Additional to the main structure (and not shown on the map) were specialist hospitals for obstetrics (Suva), tuberculosis (Tamavua), and leprosy (Makogai), and institutions privately-owned by companies or churches.

Hospital admission data are likely to be distorted in several ways. It may over-represent the population readily accessible in the immediate hinterland of the hospital, will be confined to more serious cases, and may reflect ethnic differences in attitudes to the disease.

Two of the four waves are selected for special study.

Wave III: 1910-14. The third wave is unusual, both because of its duration and its uncertain origin. No cases were recorded in 1910, but in the following year there was a major outbreak followed by a sequence of localised epidemics which appear to have persisted through to 1914.

The most dramatic incident was the introduction of measles for the first time into the island of Rotuma. The district medical officer for the island, Dr H. Macdonald, had been on leave in the early part of 1911 but returned in late March to find the outbreak in full swing:

> Measles was introduced on the 19th January when I was absent and on my return 700 cases were reported to me as existing. The epidemic continued throughout April and May and finally died out in June. It caused 50 deaths in March, 198 in April, 74 in May, and 4 in June.(19)

Macdonald calculated the death rate for the year as 246 per thousand, a five-fold increase on the 1900-10 mean for Rotuma of forty-nine. Although the exact number of deaths from measles is unclear, it probably lies between 326 (the sum for March to June) and 391 (the total deaths minus the 'expected' deaths based on the decade 1900-10 in which the island had been free from the disease). Macdonald unequivocally attributes the high rate to 'the epidemic of measles which, allowed to run through the people for the first time during my absence on leave, swept them off literally in hundreds'.(20) If we accept the mid-point of the two estimates, this would give a death rate for measles of 180 per thousand. But since his report speaks of measles being accompanied or followed by 'acute ileo-colitis' and an outbreak of influenza from late April into May, any more exact estimates are not possible. Certainly April and May are the months with the highest deaths from measles, and the continued presence of measles with influenza is known from the northern shores of the Pacific to have been a particularly virulent combination (Wolfe, 1982).

Although events in the rest of Fiji were less dramatic, they were serious enough on a local scale. Measles were present in a mild epidemic form in Suva from early February and were to continue for the rest of the year. From there it was brought on March 11 by a half-caste child into Kadavu West (186 cases and four deaths) and in early April into Labasa by the S.S. Motusa. In both areas active steps were taken to limit the spread of the disease:

> Every effort was made to stamp out the disease by isolation of the infected patient and his friends and by practically quarantining the whole village. Such disinfection as was possible was practiced but this was very limited and it was impossible to disinfect the Fijian houses except by burning down the same.(21)

Quarantining appears to have been successful; the figures for hospital admissions show little evidence of spread outside these areas.

But over the next three years measles continued to be introduced into the colony and localised epidemics were widely recorded. As the Chief Medical Officer stoically observed in his 1912 Annual Report, 'As cases of measles arrive in the colony with every immigrant ship and are sent to plantation hospitals, there must always be a few cases from time to time observed'.(22) Reports of small outbreaks from Lautaka, Labasa, and Nadi were each confined to particular estates and were largely confined to Indian children.

But inevitably spread from the estates to the rest of the island population would sometimes occur. In 1913, Dr E.G. Arnold, the District Medical Officer for Lautoka, noted a spread of cases from Nadi into the Fijian villages with 111 cases and fifteen deaths.(23) Several outbreaks were recorded at Rewa, and a major epidemic among Fijians in Colo in 1914.(24)

Wave VI: 1936-37. In January 1936, Fiji experienced its sixth major measles epidemic. The outbreak began in Suva and by the time it was complete, seventeen months later in May 1937, some 3,500 cases had been notified and 225 admitted to hospital. Despite the high attack rate, the mortality rate was practically nil with only one death due to respiratory complications of broncho-pneumonia. Dr D.W. Hoodless of the Central Medical School at Fiji noted that while Fijians had a mild attack

> Polynesians [sic] suffered severely and underwent a prolonged convalescence. Gilbertese, Ellice Islanders and Tongans seemed to be the most affected.(25)

While age data are not available, it is likely from comments in the Reports that the Fijian cases were primarily amongst children, while the Polynesians were migrant workers.

Under A.H.B. Pearce's period as Director of Medical Services the statistical content of the Annual Medical Report had been strengthened, and it is possible to gain a more precise view of the spatial distribution and course of the epidemic. The monthly totals for reported cases are disaggregated into 'Suva' and 'Country Districts'. In Suva, the epidemic lasted a bare six months with a sharp peak in April when nearly one half the cases occur. In the country districts, the epidemic lasted three times as long as in the capital city with a less pronounced peak in August.

Detailed district by month figures are not published, but it is possible to construct a rough map (Figure 8) of the progress of the epidemic. By July 1936 only the area around Suva was free of the disease while by the end of the year, all but the extreme west of Viti Levu was clear. In Vanua Levu the western part of the island was still reporting cases, as was Taveuni and Lau. In so far as evidence was available the sixth wave appeared to follow the centre-to-periphery course from Suva out to the more remote areas of the island group.

The availability of data for hospital admissions, as well as notified cases, gives an opportunity to cross check the two sources. The overall ratio of hospital admissions for measles to reported cases is 1:13 and this varies little between the two years. There is, however, more variability by geographical area. In the case of the eastern province of Lau, the rate is 1:7, and on the island of Kandavu more than 1:2. Even on the larger islands, high rates are found, as in the northern and western parts of Vanua Levu (1:4) or the Suva area of Viti Levu (1:8). The map of hospital admissions for measles gives therefore a filtered version of the incidence for the disease. It appears to be slightly higher in the capital city and very much higher in some of the outlying islands. In the rural areas of the two main islands, it is substantially higher in the predominantly Indian areas than in the predominantly Fijian.

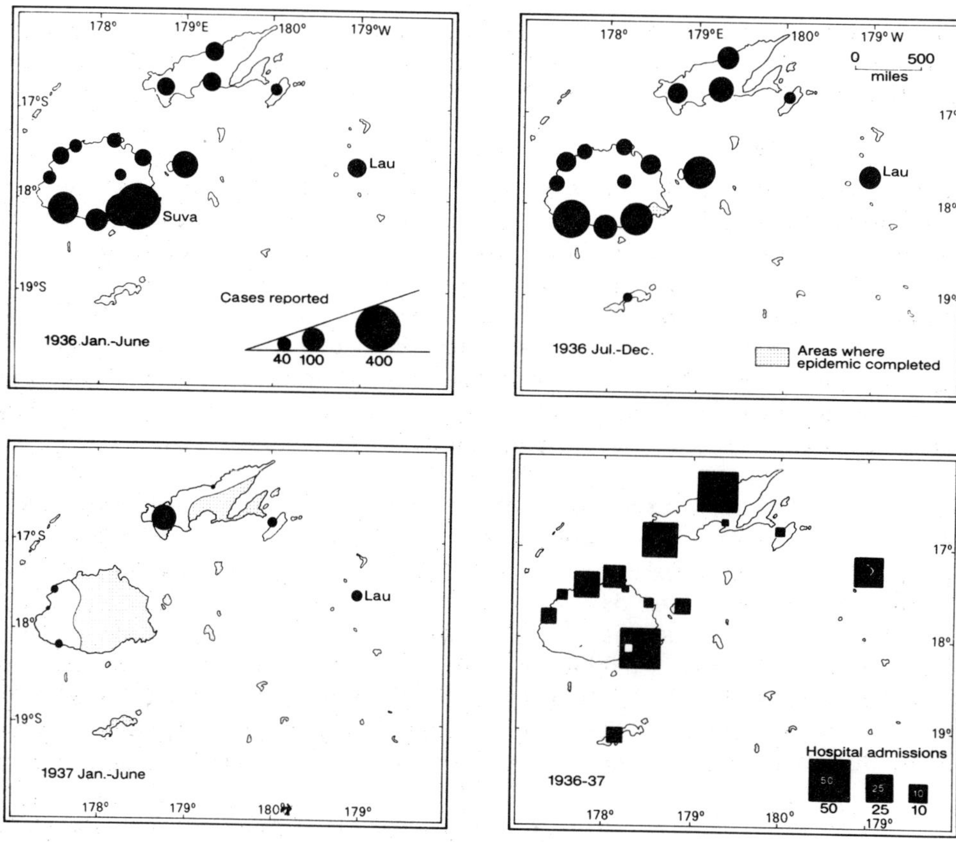

Figure 8: Measles incidence for Fiji, January 1936 - May 1937.

In the light of these comparisons it would appear that where only hospital admission data is available, these should be treated with caution. The main outlines are likely to be correct, but the regional detail may be biased both by the geographical location, hospital availability, and racial composition.

Waves VII to XIV: the evidence of case notifications

Sources of evidence. By the 1930s, an elaborate reporting mechanism had been established by which notifiable disease was reported weekly (or in certain cases, daily) to the Chief Medical Officer in Suva. This foreshadowed the present reporting system under the Public Health Ordinance by which infectious diseases are divided into three categories. In Group A are diseases (e.g. cholera) which are so serious that they must be notified immediately by telephone or telegram. In Group B are diseases (e.g. meningitis) which are notified weekly in detail by name, address, age and race. In Group C are diseases which are notified weekly in aggregate by number, race and sex. Measles, together with most of the common infectious diseases (chicken pox, dengue fever, German measles, influenza and whooping cough) falls into the last category. The precise reporting system is described in detail by Navarunisaravi (1970).

As the number of measles cases that needed hospital treatment dropped and a death from measles became a very rare event, it was the reported morbidity figures that provided evidence for epidemic waves. Two problems remained. First, the specific number of cases reported was usually an underestimate, particularly in the more remote island areas. Thus, the District Medical Officer for Savusavu notes that

> owing to the scattered nature of the district, reports of the appearance of the disease were very slow in reaching me while a great number of cases were never reported at all. No accurate figures as to the number of deaths or cases are therefore available.(26)

None the less, the officer's guess that practically the whole infant population and a large number of adults had been affected by measles in the first six months of that year leaves no doubts that a major epidemic was in progress.

Second, the published medical reports became more streamlined, and frequently only monthly totals for the colony were published. The specific regional and temporal data remained unpublished, but summaries and, for recent years, original returns are retained in the archives of the Health Department in Suva.

It is some compensation that, at a larger spatial scale, the availability of international health records improves with the advent of the Health Department of the South Pacific Commission. The Commission was set up in 1947 by the six governments then responsible for the administration of the island territories in the South Pacific. Since then the majority of the independent island countries have joined the Commission while most of the self-governing countries or dependent territories participate in the Commission programs.

Waves VII to XIV: 1945 to 1983. The published medical records for the war years are patchy since district medical officers were drafted for service elsewhere and replacements were hard to obtain. Such records as were available show no evidence of major measles epidemics. Indeed, the reports note an absence of any serious outbreaks of infectious disease of any kind.(27) This is the more surprising in view of the greatly increased sea and air contacts with Fiji which became, for two years, a major staging base in the Pacific war. As V.W.T. McGusty comments

> The Colony enjoyed a remarkable freedom from infectious diseases, although the contrary might have been expected from the presence of Armed Forces in large numbers.(28)

In this respect, Fiji was more fortunate than Papua New Guinea which experienced a number of measles outbreaks originating amongst Australian servicemen (Walker, 1957:9, 379). By 1944, the military presence in Fiji had been greatly reduced and the shipping contacts fell back to their pre-war volumes. The legacy of air-strips remained a valuable one and air traffic continued to make increasing use of Fiji as a staging post.

The detailed sequence of post-war waves is shown in Figure 9. Their characteristics are discussed in the next section.

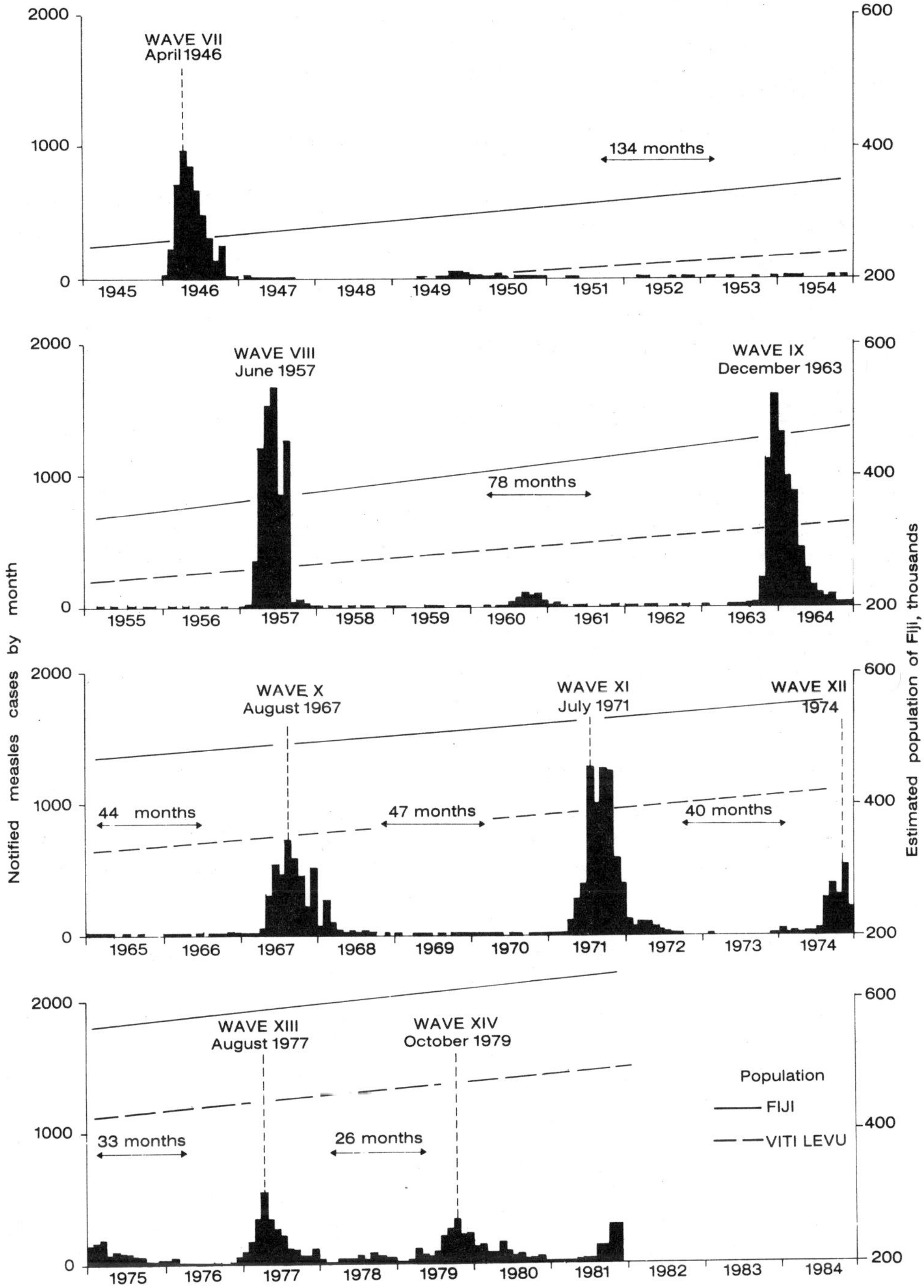

Figure 9: Monthly incidence of measles cases in Fiji for the period January 1945 onwards (Waves XIV to XIV).

NOTES

1. Sydney Gazette, 16th August 1826, p.3.

2. Sydney Gazette, 28th March 1828, p.2.

3. W.G. Lawes. Letter to Mullins, Foreign Secretary, London Missionary Society, 8 March 1875. LMS Correspondence. Cited by N. Oram, in Winslow (1977, p. 91).

4. The classic accounts of the geography of Fiji are given in Ward (1965) and Brookfield and Hart (1971).

5. Report of the Commission, etc., op.cit.

6. Letter from the Admiralty to Commodore Hawkins conveying their views on the alleged introduction of measles into Fiji by the officers of HMS Dido. British Parliamentary Papers. Accounts and Papers. 1876 (399). LIV.237.

7. Fiji Argus, Levuka, March 19th 1875.

8. To Colonial Secretary, Fiji, 27 October, C.S.O. (Inwards) 87/2851. Cited by Joyce, (1971, p.25).

9. One of the fullest accounts is given in Report of the Commission appointed to inquire into the decrease of the native population. Suva, Colony of Fiji, 1896. See also the official reports recorded in Parliamentary papers (C1634).

10. Fiji Times, Levuka, Wednesday December 13th, 1875, p.5.

11. Much of the substance of the official reports on the 1875 outbreak is concerned with 'buck-passing' between the authorities directly involved. See references cited in McArthur (1967).

12. Fiji Argus, Levuka, 20th April 1875.

13. Fiji, Colonial Secretary's Office. Inward correspondence. Letter from Dr McGregor, 7th September 1875.

14. Idem. 8th September 1875.

15. The Times, London, 9th June 1875, p.5.

16. Public Health Board. *Regulations by the Board of Health in view of the presence of Measles in the Colony.* *Fiji Legislative Council Paper*, No.21, 18th September 1893.

17. G.W.A. Lynch, Chief Medical Officer, 13 May 1913. *Annual Medical Report, 1913.* Fiji. Legislative Council Paper, No.32, 1913, p.13.

18. A. Montague, Chief Medical Officer, 24 May 1922. *Annual Medical Report for the year ending 31st December 1921.* *Fiji. Legislative Council Paper*, No.51, 1922. Suva, 1923, p.4.

19. H. Macdonald, Rotuma Medical District, in G.W.A. Lynch, Chief Medical Officer, *Annual Medical Report for 1911.* Fiji. Legislative Council Paper, No.32, 1912, p.20.

20. Macdonald, op.cit., p.20.

21. Report by District Medical Officer for Kadavu. In *Annual Medical Report for 1911.* op.cit., p.12.

22. G.W.A. Lynch, Chief Medical officer, *Annual Medical Report, 1912.* Fiji. Legislative Council Paper, No.32, 1913, p.13.

23. E.G. Arnold. District Medical Report for Lautoka. In *Annual Medical Report, 1913.* Fiji. Legislative Council Paper, No.44, 1914, p.13.

24. A. Montague, Chief Medical Officer, *Annual Medical Report, 1914.* Fiji. Legislative Council Paper, No.23, 1915, p.4.

25. In A.H.B. Pearce, Chief Medical Officer, *Annual Medical and Health Report for 1936.* Fiji. Legislative Council Paper, No.27, 1937, p.33. It is worth noting that in fact the Gilbertese are Micronesian. Ellice Islanders are Polynesian. One problem is that in Fiji in the nineteenth and early twentieth centuries the term 'Polynesian' was often applied to islanders from any other part of the Pacific, and especially those from Melanesia. Most of the so-called 'Polynesian' indentured labourers in Fiji were in fact from Melanesia (New Hebrides and Solomons mainly).

26. W.E. Hallinan, District Report for Savusavu. *Annual Medical Report for the year ending 31st December 1921.* Fiji. Legislative Council Paper, No.51, 1922 Sessions.

Suva, 1923, p.17.

27. D.C. Macpherson, Chief Medical Officer, Annual Medical Report, 1940. Fiji Legislative Council Paper, No.5, 1941, p.6.

28. V.W.T. McGusty, Chief Medical Officer, Annual Medical Report, 1943. Fiji Legislative Council Paper, 1944, p.3.

CHAPTER 3

SPATIAL ANALYSIS

THE WAVE SEQUENCES: AN ISLAND PERSPECTIVE

The sequence of waves described for the Fijian group in the previous chapter raises a number of questions about the transmission of diseases in island groups. We look at these first at the level of Fiji itself (the 'island' perspective) and then in the context of the wider region (the 'Pacific' perspective). We raise here three such questions at the island scale relating to (1) mortality, (2) sources of infection, and (3) intervention in the spread process.

Mortality

The death rate from the initial Fijian wave was of awful proportions: the various estimates are discussed above and in further demographic detail by McArthur (1967). Even if one takes a conservative estimate, the losses in the first half of 1875 amounted to more than one in five of the Fijian native population.

The demographic impact of contemporary measles outbreaks on 'virgin soil' (i.e. previously unexposed) populations has been widely studied. See, for example, the work of F.L. Black and others (Black, 1976; Black et al., 1977; Black and Rosen, 1962; Christensen et al., 1953; Peart and Nagler, 1954). Notwithstanding these remarks, one of the fullest and earliest accounts of deaths in a measles epidemic was Peter Panum's description of the experience of the Faeroes Islands' population in 1846 (Panum, 1940). The sixty-five year gap since the last epidemic of 1781 meant that the greater part of the population could be regarded as 'virgin soil' in terms of measles susceptibility. From Panum's detailed figures, a death rate from measles of 23 per 1000 is indicated. This is about four times the normal death rate in the Faeroes at that period and was mainly made up by an excess of deaths in the infant and 60-65 year age group.

TABLE 4: ESTIMATED DEATH RATE FROM MEASLES IN ISOLATED POPULATIONS

Year	Location	Years since previous outbreak	Number of deaths on which rate estimated	Estimated death rate per thousand
A 1846	Faeroe Islands	65 (1781)	180	23
B 1846	Iceland	58 (1788)	107	39
C 1860-61	Western Aust.	57	57	2
D 1875	Fiji	'Virgin soil'	c.40,000	250
E 1882	Iceland	36 (1846)	250	45
F 1900	Alaska	W. Alaska: 'Virgin soil' Aleutians: ?25 (1875)	1,000+	c.250
G 1903	Fiji	28 (1875)	c.2,000	?
H 1952+	Americas	'Virgin soil'	?	30-270

For definition of 'virgin soil' populations, see text.

Sources: (A) Panum (1940) Deaths mainly amongst infants and 60-65 years. (B) Cliff et al. (1983) Mortality rate for Reykjavik area only. (C) Cumpston (1927) immigrant European population; first major outbreak in colony. (D) See details in this paper. (E) Cliff et al. (1983) Mortality rate for N.W. Iceland only. (F) Wolfe (1982) Conjoint measles + influenza epidemic; deaths mainly amongst Aleut, Eskimo and Indian populations; Europeans unaffected. (G) See details in this paper. (H) Black (1976) Isolated American Indian tribes; death rates vary from 30-96 for N. American to 180-270 for S. American.

As Table 4 indicates, the death rate from measles outbreaks in virgin-soil populations is high. But the Fijian mortality appears to be higher in comparison with other measles epidemics, so that some special explanation might need to be looked for. Three factors may well have multiplied up the expected deaths.

First is the sheer scale of the outbreak. It seems likely that more than 100,000 people were affected by the virus, all within a span of six months. The breakdown of 'normal' life in terms of food gathering and hygiene, plus the contagious fear of a new affliction whose duration and outcome were unknown, all exacerbated the effects. The prevalence of dysentry and the lack of care for the very young, the very old and the sick are all documented. Even those who were medically fit were so bowed down by the scale of the disaster that they ceased to care for their own health.

A second factor was undoubtedly due to the 'treatment' exacerbating the initial problem. The 1896 commission reports that

> One correspondent relates that during the epidemic of measles, in 1875, natives persisted in trying to cool their fevered bodies by lying for hours in the water and in damp places, in spite of strict orders to the contrary. A child heated with fever is plunged into cold water or set naked in the breeze or damp grass to cool its body. Such ignorance...is to be expected among a people lately confronted with diseases unknown to their fathers and whose knowledge of diseases is solely derived from empiricism.(1)

How widespread the practice was is unknown, but it was still being resorted to sixteen years later during the 1891-92 influenza epidemic.

Where normal rest and nursing was available, the death rate was much lower. In the Nadi area of Viti Levu, the local JP circulated pamphlets on 'what to do and what to avoid if taken with the disease' to head teachers and village chiefs. He reports only eleven deaths in eight or ten villages with a population of more than 2,000 and suggested similarly low figures were typical of the imported labourers who were also following standard instructions.(2)

The overlap of the measles epidemic with an unusually severe hurricane season may well have intensified the general health problems in the early part of 1875. An 'Occasional Correspondent' wrote from Levuka on April 23 to <u>The Times</u>:

> The ravages of the epidemic have been necessarily extended by reason of the unfortunate time of the

> year at which it was communicated. You will have observed that it was introduced...in January, the commencement of which is termed the hurricane season - the most inclement of the year.(3)

This particular season was apparently an unusually severe one for the correspondent goes on

> This year it has visited with exceptional severity. On the 8th January the islands encountered a terrific gale of wind, accompanied by downpour of rain in torrents; and from that time until the end of the last month [March] the weather has been almost unknown. The 'oldest inhabitant' declares there has never been so dreadful a time. Certainly for the last 16 years there has been experienced no such weather, and nothing could be more fatal to a diseased Fijian than exposure to it.(4)

It seems evident that in the early months of 1875, little would go right for the Fijian people.

The high mortality in the first three waves stands in stark contrast to that of waves in the rest of this century (Table 3). The reasons behind the decline are complex. As Silvester-Evans comments in his 1946 report:

> It would appear that an enhanced resistance has developed in the indigenous Fijian population...It is true that the course of the [1946] epidemic is reflected in the increase in crude death rate and the infant and child mortality rates, but taken by and large measles has lost some of the terror it previously held as a killing disease in the islands. How much that is due to increased resistance, how much to improved environmental conditions, and how much to an increased knowledge of what not to do with any febrile ailment in children is for deliberate consideration in the light of future events.(5)

Such future events have continued the steady fall in the mortality of measles and its complications.

Geographical sources of infection

With the establishment of British rule, detailed port statistics begin to be assembled and the contacts between Fiji and outside source areas can be measured.(6) Records for 1876, the year following the first epidemic, show that sixty-one foreign vessels called into Fiji. Comparison of these statistics with the report of vessels arriving in 1875 given in the Fiji Times and the Fiji Argus show a broadly similar pattern. The leading source area was New South Wales (fourteen vessels), followed by New Zealand (thirteen), New Hebrides (nine) and Tonga (seven). No other area had more than five vessels and these came from other Pacific Island groups (Samoa, Rotuma, Line Islands, and the Solomons), with a single ship coming directly from England. From the viewpoint of disease spread, the number of people on each ship may be a more relevant parameter than a count of ships. A history of crew numbers is available and shows a total of 520, an average of between eight or nine on each vessel. Ships sailing the longer routes tended to be the larger and this increases the relative importance of New South Wales as a source area from around 23 per cent to 30 per cent.

Customs records(7) for the three ports handling foreign vessels - Levuka, Suva and Lomaloma - show that vessels were overwhelmingly heading for Levuka. Whether measured by the value of imports or of customs dues, over 97 per cent of traffic was concentrated onto the island of Ovalau in 1876. It was therefore, an obvious point of entry for foreign diseases at that time. With the shift of the capital to Suva on Viti Levu, the focus of importation shifted and the role of Levuka rapidly diminished. Lomaloma ceased to be a port of entry.

For the early outbreaks three sources of infection appear to be important - Australia, New Zealand and India. Each is reviewed in turn.

Australia as a source. Australia in general and New South Wales in particular was the leading potential source of measles virus for Fiji. As Figure 10 shows, deaths from measles were recorded continuously from 1850 and Australia may reasonably be regarded as a reservoir for the virus from that date. It was also the major trading partner for Fiji and the average sailing time of three weeks was well within two generations of the virus.

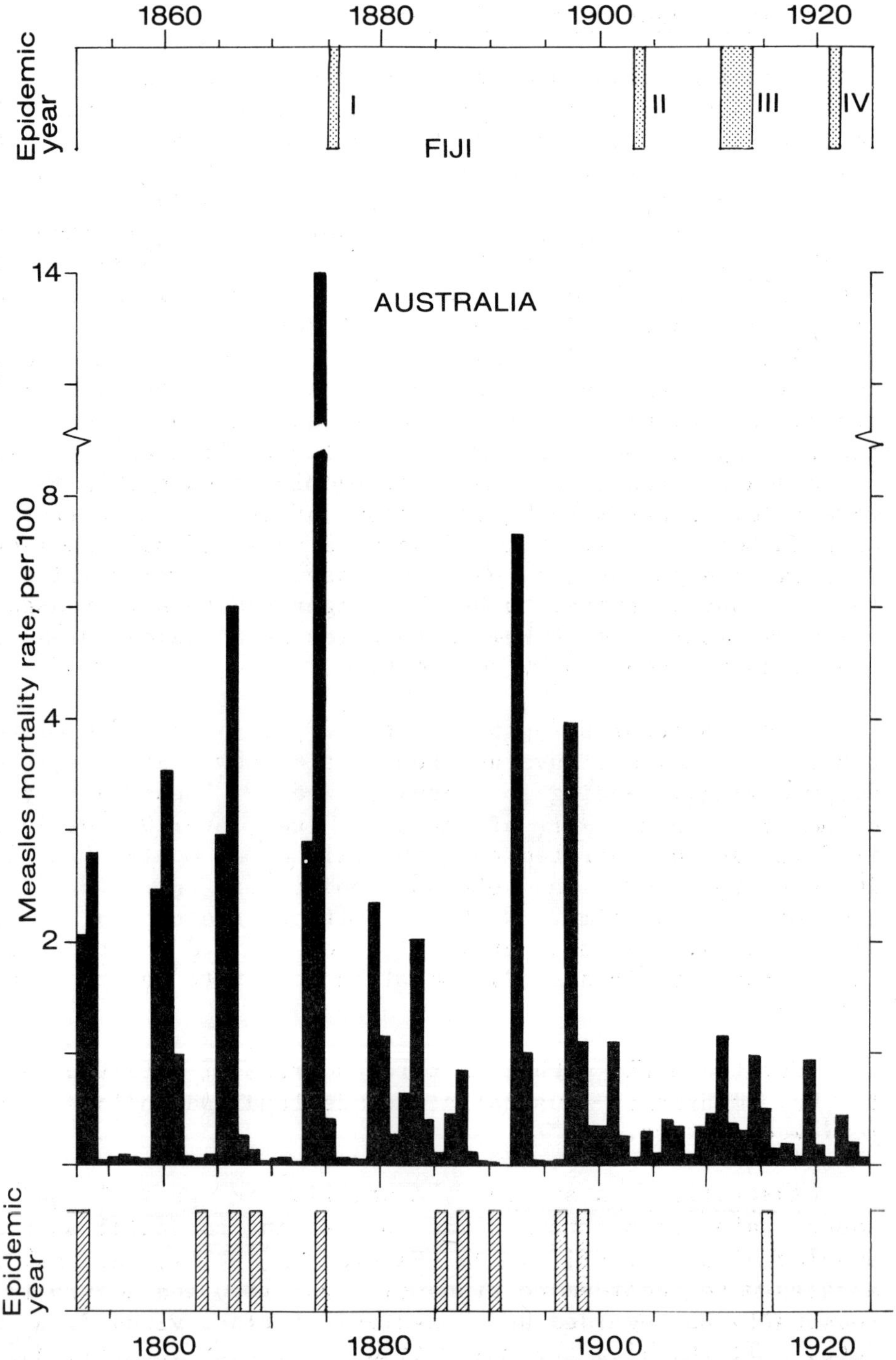

Figure 10: Death rate from measles in Australia, 1852-1924.

The unequivocal link from Australia to Fiji in 1875 has already been discussed at length in our examination of that Fijian epidemic. The first four Fijian waves appear as the top part of Figure 10 but, apart from the first, there is no direct evidence for a further Australian introduction in this period. The sources of the subsequent waves are not known, but since Australian ports were a dominant origin for foreign ships calling at the main Fijian ports at this time, they may well have proved an important reservoir of infection. The absence of Australian morbidity records for measles (apart from South Australia where measles was a notifiable disease) is particularly frustrating in this respect.

Although it is not our direct concern, it is interesting to note that work has been done on sources of infection for Australia itself. Thus, the possible links between major measles epidemics in England and Wales and Australia have been investigated at length by Cumpston (1927) using the records of ships arriving at the main Australian ports. Although measles in England and Wales settled down to a regular three-yearly cycle, in Australia the mortality records (Figure 10) show great variation with peaks at irregular intervals of five years and more. While there is some visual correspondence between major epidemic years in both regions, it would be difficult to establish any virological foundation for such an association. Cumpston (1927:258) suggests that the course of measles epidemics in Australia may be affected by 'fresh infections introduced at intervals, which superimposed upon the course of the disease in Australia the complications of a new strain of virus with a new starting point in the time cycle'. There are two difficulties with Cumpston's hypothesis. First, the idea of 'new strains' is not substantiated by subsequent work on measles which suggests that the measles virus -- unlike influenza -- is genetically stable. Second, the direct link to English ports ignores the possible epidemiological role of intermediate stops along the route; for example, the link to conditions in the Cape Colony of southern Africa remains an intriguing one.(8) If European or African populations there were infected, they would serve as an important booster for new cases to be carried on to Australia.

New Zealand as a source. The role of New Zealand as a source area is even less well documented that that of Australia. Although measles was known to be raging in New Zealand in 1875(9), this was probably a secondary infection from Australia. The first reference to cases imported from

New Zealand occurs in 1918(10), and there are sporadic references during the inter-war years. In most cases the index case is European and a child. One typical case occurred in 1920:

> In December [1920] a case was imported from New Zealand, where the disease was rife by children coming back from school and a small epidemic was started of a very mild type.(11)

Although New Zealand's role was a secondary one to Australia in the earlier period, the growing links between Fiji and Auckland in the last half century have probably increased its relative importance as an infection source.

India as a source. The history of Indian migration to Fiji up to the end of indenture in 1920 has been extensively studied by Gillion (1962). Over the thirty-seven years between 1879 and 1916, Indian immigrant ships made eighty-seven voyages to Fiji carrying nearly 61,000 indentured emigrants. The health and welfare of the immigrants were the responsibility of the Surgeon-Superintendent who accompanied each ship and whose report was incorporated into the *Annual Reports on Indian Immigration* published regularly as *Official Papers of Fiji's Legislative Council.*

From these reports, the presence of measles can be detected and the link to Fijian epidemics traced. For example, the 1911 Report records 'many cases of measles breaking out' on the *Mutlah* and 'an epidemic of measles of a mild type' on the *Sutlej*, but the other three voyages in the second half of the year were free of that disease.(12) Usually, the incidence of the disease was broken down by age and sex in the records. Thus, the 1901 report records that

> The outbreak of measles on board the *Fazilka* appears to have been of a severe type. There were 44 cases, 15 males, 10 females, 7 boys, 6 girls, 4 male infants and 2 female infants. Of these 2 men and 2 women died on the voyage. 2 patients landed in the Colony and died in hospital.(13)

Since measles was endemic in much of India, it was not surprising that cases should be recorded although there were checks in the camps both at Calcutta and Madras, the two exit ports, before embarkation. Figure 11, which has been constructed from the evidence in the Fijian annual reports,

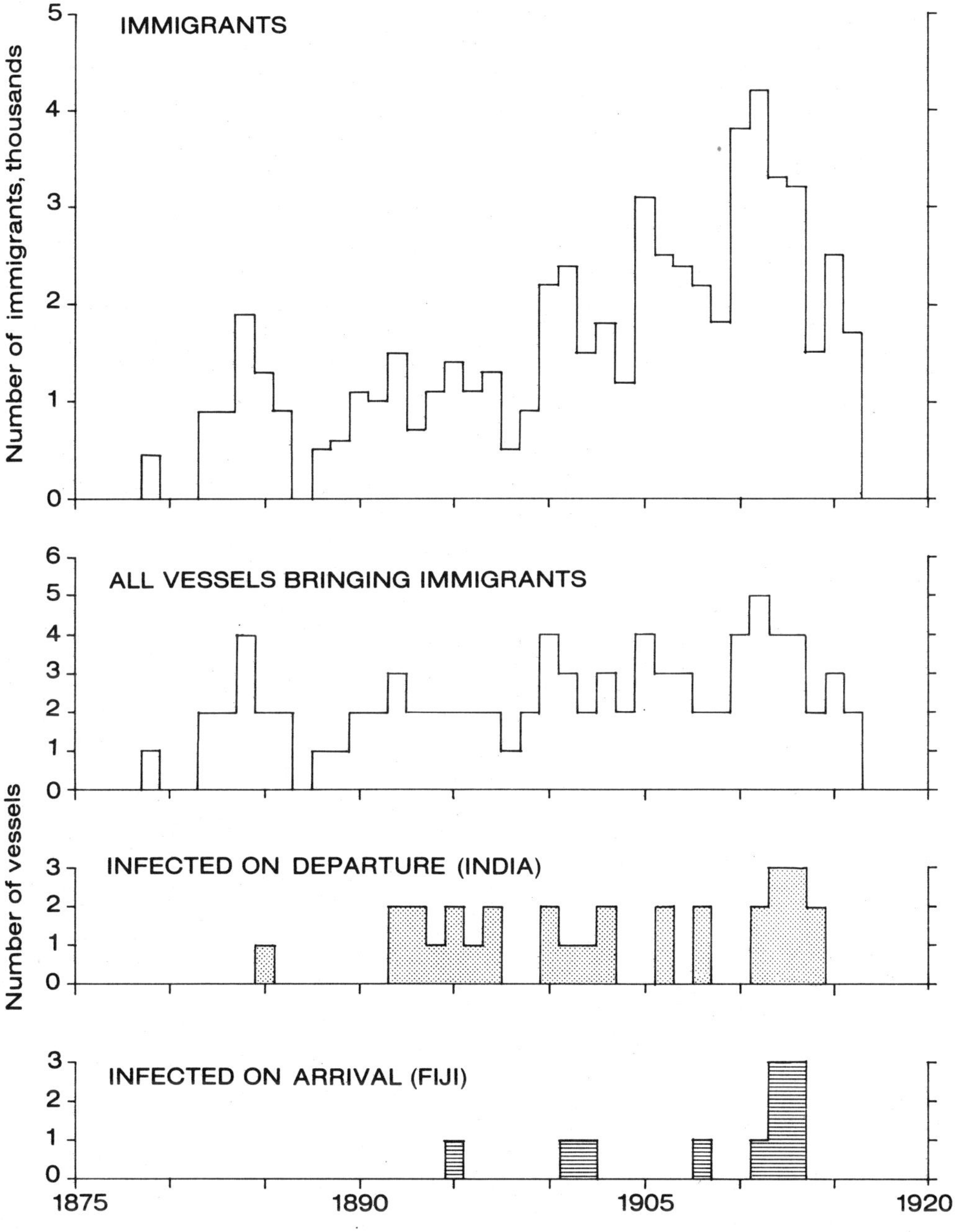

Figure 11: Vessels carrying indentured immigrants between India and Fiji from 1879 through 1916.

show that measles was detected on board during thirty-two of the voyages. These are broadly distributed over time and reflect the 1:3 probability of being infected on departure from India.

Figure 11 goes on to show, using data collected from the same source, the distribution of voyages where vessels were still infected with measles on arrival in Fiji. These amount to only eleven, indicating that measles did not survive in two-thirds of the voyages in which it was known to be present. Such voyages all occur late in the emigration period. The explosive growth of a measles epidemic is illustrated by a subsequent voyage of the _Fazilka_ in 1903. In this instance, two cases were reported in the first half of the voyage, eight in the second half, but 130 in the quarantine depot at Nukulau Island within ten days of landing.(14)

Some of the factors behind this distribution of infected arrivals are shown in Figure 12. This plots each voyage in terms of its length in days and the size of the vessel. Clearly, an important distinction must be drawn between the sailing ships used between 1879 and 1904 and the steamships used between 1884 and 1916. Sailing ships followed the route south of Australia and took about seventy days for the voyage. Steamships came through the Torres Strait north of Australia and halved the sailing ship times; they were also able to carry a larger number of immigrants. The threat of speeding the introduction of measles into Fiji by using the faster and larger steamships was considered by the medical officers on the ships, but they did not rate the risk as critical:

> so far as can be judged as yet the introduction of immigrants by steamers has not had a prejudicial effect on their health, though it increases the chance of introducing diseases of a severe type into the colony and renders more likely the necessity of imposing quarantine.(15)

For the virus to persist in a steamship voyage it needed only two, or at most three, generations of measles attacks, assuming an average link length of fourteen days (Figure 2). On the sailing ships, virus persistence required five or six generations, and this within a slightly smaller population of passengers. It is not surprising that it was the steamships, rather than sailing ships, which brought measles from India.

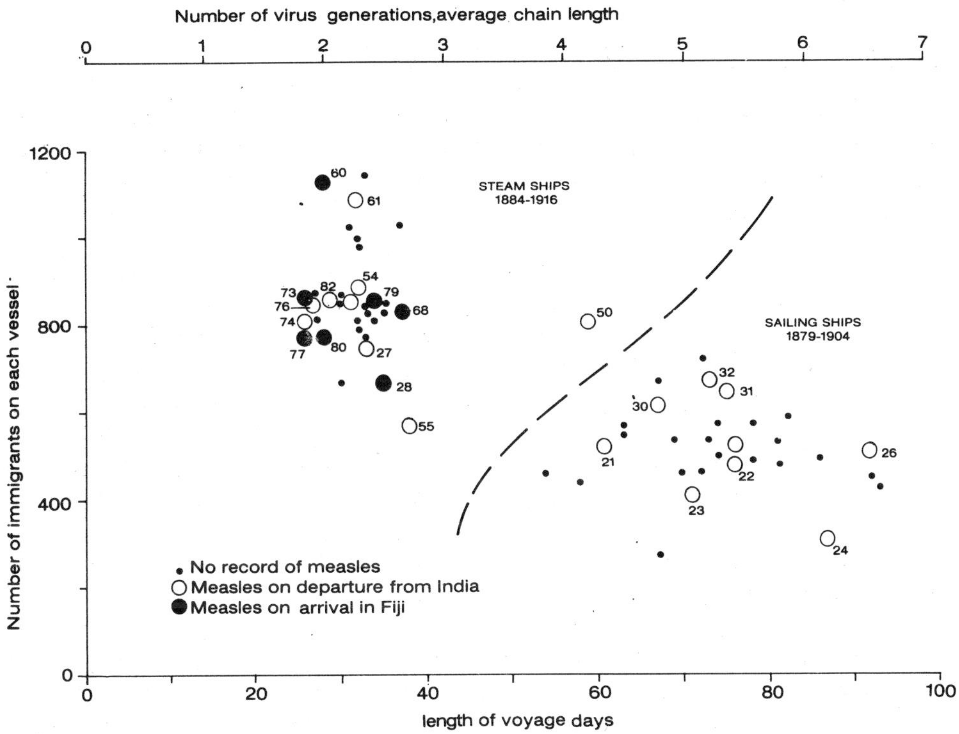

Figure 12: Vessels carrying indentured immigrants between India and Fiji, 1879 to 1916.

Even amongst those ships arriving with measles on board, the chance of starting an epidemic on Fiji itself was quite small. One factor was that all immigrant ships were quarantined and inspected on arrival. The first quarantine station was established on Yamuca Levu island between Ovalau and Moturiki islands and was used by the first immigrants from the Leonidas. With the shift of the Fijian capital to Suva, the quarantine station was moved to the island of Nukulau on the reef about 10 km east of Suva harbour. Immigrants were usually detained for a fourteen day period before being delivered to the plantation areas.

A second factor limiting the spread of measles was that an infected migrant (usually a child) would be joining an Indian plantation community in which most Indians would have a natural immunity due to previous infection. The proportion of susceptibles in the locally infected community was therefore low.

Intervention in the spread process

The idea of a native people passively accepting the diffusion of an unwelcome disease is inherently an unlikely one. Isolation and quarantine were in no sense new or wholly European ideas:

> The occurrence of infectious illnesses strange to the Fijians was soon associated with the presence of strangers and prior to the acceptance of Christianity the recognized method of imposing quarantine regulations was by 'club law'.(16)

One of the earliest references to its application in the South Pacific in the case of measles was in May 1851. On Eromanga, the Rev. G.H.N. Gordon and his wife were killed by the natives in consequence of an outbreak of measles which had been introduced by a trading vessel.(17)

Much of the official correspondence and inquiry which followed the fatal 1875 outbreak was concerned with quarantine law and the failure of H.M.S. *Dido* to fly the yellow flag on entering Levuka harbour. But in January 1875, there was no quarantine law in Fiji and the quarantine code for New South Wales was not introduced until late in the following month. By that time, the case for quarantine was long past: as Thurston wrote 'people talk of isolation. They might as well talk of setting a barricade against the east wind'.(18)

The imposition of strict quarantine from 1875 onwards was kept up by the first two chief medical officers for thirty years, then progressively abandoned. The changing views of the value of quarantine were reflected by Fiji's chief medical officer in 1922. Noting the catastrophic epidemic of 1875 he observed that

> As a result careful quarantine was unfortunately maintained against the disease and it was kept out until 1903...since then no special measures have

> been taken and several localized epidemics have occurred...but the death rate has been very low.(19)

He concludes from the evidence of 1903 (see the earlier description of Wave II) that it would be unwise to exclude the disease and thus produce an adult non-immune population.

Montague's rather modern views of the epidemiology of measles and the relative balance of deaths were not universally shared. Quarantining of Indian passengers on immigrant boats was routine up to 1916 and a special isolation centre was built for that purpose. In addition, at the local level, his own District Medical Officers worked hard to prevent the spread of the disease. Thus, in 1928, the report for Nadroga spoke of an outbreak being prevented from spreading by 'strict isolation and disinfecting'.(20) There appeared, therefore, to be some inconsistency between views of isolation at the colony-wide and the local level.

By the 1960s, opinion had firmly shifted towards a non-intervention policy at both levels. Dr C.H. Gurd, the Director of Medical Services, commented in his 1963 report that

> The repeated introduction of the disease safeguards the population against high mortality rates such as occur when the disease is introduced to populations which are unfamiliar with the disease.(21)

and again in the 1967 report

> It is considered good public health practice not to try and prevent this natural immunity being acquired by the children of Fiji.(22)

By the latter date a wholly new type of intervention was beginning to be available, namely vaccination.

Live vaccine from attenuated measles virus was developed and tested by J.F. Enders and his associates in 1958. This vaccine was licensed for manufacture in the United States in 1963. Its widespread use there since 1965 has had a dramatic effect on measles incidence and by late 1983, the Centers for Disease Control (CDC) estimated that 'endemic' measles (as opposed to secondary cases arising from imported measles) had been effectively eliminated from the continental United States. A small number of cases continue to be recorded from infected individuals entering the United States, especially from Mexico. For the Pacific, the success of the American vaccination campaign can be best seen in Hawaii and is referred to in the next section.

Vaccination remains expensive and the dangers of larger numbers of adults being infected in rare but major epidemics in a partially vaccinated population continue. The official view in Fiji when the vaccine first became available that 'the expense and trouble of measles immunisation is not justified at present'(23) is being reviewed. Despite the demonstration that, in developed countries, the costs of vaccination are outweighed fourfold by the benefits (Ambrosch, Wiederman and Harasek, 1978), the problem remains, for many small Pacific countries, more an economic than a strictly medical one. It may take a global campaign, on the lines argued by Hinman and his associates at CDC, before elimination of the measles virus from the Pacific populations would be forseeable. Medical opinion is divided and it would be dangerous and misleading to draw analogies with smallpox; however, a substantial reduction in measles incidence through immunization in the Pacific is forseeable and achievable.

THE WAVE SEQUENCE: A PACIFIC PERSPECTIVE

By combing published source materials in the World Health Organization's papers, in the records available in the Australian Department of Health Library at Woden, and in the archives of the Australian National Library, an incomplete sequence of monthly records for some twenty Pacific countries can be built up. A useful review of the medical literature for the southwest Pacific is provided by Norman-Taylor (1963-78). The resulting data matrix is summarised in Table 5 and Figure 13A. Here the records are arranged in a monthly sequence (from January 1946 to December 1981) and by countries, from that with the fullest record to that with the most incomplete. The countries range from Fiji, with a complete record, to Norfolk Island where published data are available for only nine per cent of the time. Two countries with records, but with no recorded cases, Pitcairn and Tokelau, were eliminated from further study.

It should be noted that countries which either separated or joined together during the thirty-six year study period are treated in the analysis which follows as single units. Thus, Papua and New Guinea (which joined together in 1973) and

Kiribati and Tuvalu (which separated in 1975) are single rows in the matrix made up of the conjoint series from their two parts.

TABLE 5: SUMMARY OF MEASLES DATA FOR THE PACIFIC FROM JANUARY 1946 TO DECEMBER 1981

No.	Location	Months with measles records (max.432)	Total measles cases recorded 1946-81	Average cases per month	Average annual measles rate per 1000 population
1.	American Samoa	360	3,947	11	5.8
2.	Cook Islands	286	6,310	22	17.3
3.	Fiji	432	41,518	97	2.6
4.	French Polynesia	387	17,944	46	5.2
5.	Kiribati and Tuvalu[a]	286	20,548	72	17.4
6.	Guam	333	3,945	12	1.9
7.	Hawaii	348	41,257	119	2.2
8.	Nauru	235	889	4	9.6
9.	New Caledonia	324	7,804	24	2.9
10.	Vanuatu	262	2,461	9	1.6
11.	Niue	191	1,438	8	20.3
12.	Norfolk Island	46	267	6	36.9
13.	Papua New Guinea[b]	281	76,852	273	1.3
14.	Pitcairn	45	0	0	0.0
15.	Solomons	259	8,081	31	2.2
16.	Tokelau	48	0	0	0.0
17.	Tonga	295	17,347	59	10.3
18.	TTP[c]	360	10,856	30	3.9
19.	Wallis and Futuna	286	4,246	15	20.2
20.	Western Samoa	300	7,307	24	2.4
	Overall Pacific	268	273,017	1,019	4.6

a From 1975, the Gilbert and Ellice Islands are separate states but their records are combined for continuity of analysis.

b From 1973, Papua New Guinea are joined and their records are combined throughout the study period.

c Trust Territories of the Pacific.

TABLE 5 (contd)

No.	Location	Average cross-correlation value[d]		Average lead or lag in months of maximum cross-correlation value[e]		Largest single number in a month
		Time 1	Time 2	Time 1	Time 2	
1.	Amer. Samoa	369	419	7.6	7.1	325
2.	Cook Is.	336	-	6.1	-	2,513
3.	Fiji	332	499	7.3	9.1	1,665
4.	French Polynesia	66	554	8.3	8.2	1,867
5.	Kiribati & Tuvalu	366	426	6.6	8.5	2,500
6.	Guam	216	443	12.3	7.3	173
7.	Hawaii	290	414	7.6	9.5	2,121
8.	Nauru	-	-	-	-	65
9.	New Caledonia	238	311	13.6	7.9	646
10.	Vanuatu	313	-	10.4	-	140
11.	Niue	-	-	-	-	133
12.	Norfolk Is.	-	-	-	-	115
13.	Papua N.G.	-	246	-	7.7	1,716
14.	Pitcairn	*	*	*	*	0
15.	Solomons	264	-	12.8	-	894
16.	Tokelau	*	*	*	*	0
17.	Tonga	365	313	7.2	8.5	3,520
18.	TTP	188	381	10.2	7.4	1,852
19.	Wallis & Futuna	-	269	-	7.8	760
20.	Wes. Samoa	257	403	8.6	6.1	337
Overall Pacific		277	390	9.1	7.9	3,520

d Average of the maximum cross-correlation value (x 1000) with other locations within a period of +12 and -12 months.

e Average lead or lag in months of the maximum cross-correlation value with other locations within a period of +18 and -18 months.

* Not computable.

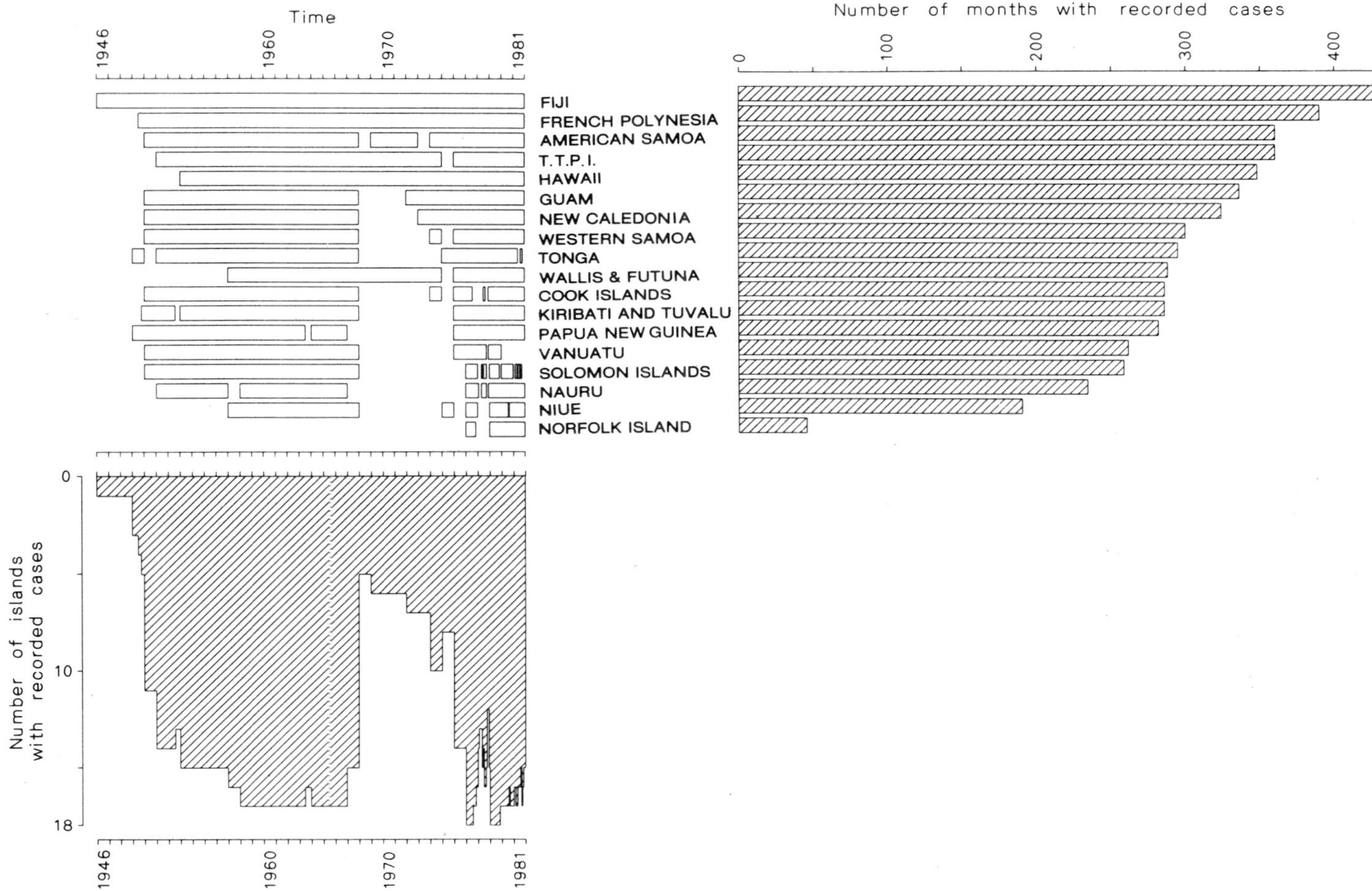

Figure 13: Availability of published data on measles incidence for twenty Pacific basin countries over the period 1946 to 1981 inclusive

The measles time series: standardisation

It is clear from the discussion of the Fiji records that the number of measles cases recorded in a particular Pacific country cannot be accepted at face value. Such numbers will reflect the quality of the local reporting network (for example, the number and location of medical practitioners) at a given time as well as the 'real' level of measles cases. Even where records exist, they are rarely complete, as Figure 13 shows. None the less, the high rate of measles incidence once an attack occurs ensures a very strong signal in the records and the difference between epidemic and non-epidemic periods is rarely ambiguous.

One approach to the standardisation of morbidity data for a series of countries with incomplete data sets is shown as a flow diagram in Figure 14. The original inputs are the recorded number of cases for each time period, t, (usually for each calendar month but for some countries as a four week period) for each country, i. To provide a more useful and consistent measure, the following steps are necessary.

(a) The number of recorded cases is converted to a monthly prevalence rate per 1,000 population by dividing through by the population of the recording country. Since population estimates are usually only available for mid-year or census points, linear interpolation to give a monthly population is also required.

(b) Prevalence rates will reflect not only (i) genuine variations in virus activity but also (ii) artificial variations in the collecting rate characteristic of a particular country. To reduce the role of (ii), the monthly prevalence rate for a country can be converted to a prevalence index by subtracting some average value and dividing by some measure of range. Given the highly skewed nature of measles records, with many cases concentrated into a few months, logarithms may first be taken to produce term (3) of Figure 14. The skewness problem is further mitigated by using the median and inter-quartile range, rather than the mean and standard deviation, as the measures of centrality and spread. This normalisation yields term (4) of Figure 14. This prevalence index allows a more meaningful comparison to be made between the epidemic histories of different countries.

Raw figures

x_{it}

↓

COMPUTE LOCAL RATE PER 1000 RESIDENT POPULATION

$$x'_{it} = 1000 \frac{x_{it}}{\text{population}_{it}}$$

↓

REDUCE THE EFFECT OF EXTREME VALUES ON THE AVERAGE OR MEDIAN

$$x''_{it} = \log(1 + x'_{it})$$

NORMALISE EACH VALUE USING AN APPROPRIATE MEASURE OF THE CENTRAL LOCATION AND RANGE OF $\{x''_i\}$) VALUES OVER t TO REFLECT LOCAL REPORTING PATTERN

$$x'''_{it} = \frac{x''_{it} - \begin{cases}\text{median} \\ \text{mean}\end{cases}(x''_i)}{\begin{cases}\text{inter-quartile range} \\ \text{standard deviation}\end{cases}(x''_i)}$$

WEIGHT OF THE NORMALISED VALUE BY THE POPULATION SIZE OF THE AREAS

↓

$$x''''_{it} = f(\text{population}_{it})\, x'''_{it}\,; \qquad x''''_{jt} = (\text{population}_{jt})\, x'''_{jt}$$

COMBINE SUFFICIENT VALUES FROM GEOGRAPHICALLY ADJACENT AREAS TO ENSURE THAT THE WEIGHTED REGIONAL AVERAGE (R) FORMS A CONTINUOUS TIME SERIES

$$x_{Rt} = \frac{(x''''_{it} + x''''_{jt} + \ldots + \ldots)}{f(\text{population}_{it}) + f(\text{population}_{jt}) + \ldots)}$$

CHECK FOR STATIONARITY IN THE WEIGHTED REGIONAL AVERAGE AND ADJUST ACCORDINGLY USING AN APPROPRIATE MONOTONIC ESTIMATING FUNCTION ($\hat{x}_{Rt}$) IF STRONG TREND

$$x'_{Rt} = \frac{x_{Rt} - \hat{x}_{Rt}}{\hat{x}_{Rt}}$$

Figure 14: Procedure for standardising incomplete time series of measles morbidity rates.

(c) The local prevalence index for a particular country is sometimes incomplete for the period of interest, with missing years or months. Complete series can sometimes be constructed by combining the series of two or more countries to give a composite or regional value. The criteria for combination may be geographical adjacency, common epidemiological history (based on the correlation of the common parts of the reduced series), or the degree of compensating overlap between two or more series. A composite series could be constructed by a simple averaging process, but in epidemiological studies of countries of varying population sizes, it would seem appropriate to consider taking this magnitude factor into account and construct term (5) of Figure 14. Several methods could be argued for; in Figure 14, the square root of the population of the member units is suggested which retains population weight, but in a reduced form. This gives term (6) of Figure 14.

(d) The composite index may be regarded as a generalised indicator of the pattern of measles activity, rather than a precise measure. On theoretical grounds, we should expect the index to reflect the known features of measles series. Where the index increases steadily over time, then we would surmise that these are due to an artificial increase in the reporting rate brought about by an increase in the number of medically qualified personnel or improved public health administration. Improved transport and increased contact are unlikely to lead to an upward trend over the long-term but rather to the substitution of smaller but more frequent peaks for larger and more widely-spaced ones. To guard against this reporting effect, the index could be conservatively estimated as residuals (term 7 of Figure 14) from a stationary trend line as given by a linear regression equation.

The measles time series: results

The sequences of measles cases for the thirty-six year period from January 1946 to December 1981 are shown in Figure 15 for the fourteen island systems with reasonably complete records. The values have been standardised following the procedures outlined above and summarised in Figure 14. Note that the main epidemics (shaded) are defined by rates which are more than one inter-quartile range (IQR) above the median for each series. Where the graphs have been constructed from the data which are given only for three- or six-monthly periods, rather than for single months, then the average

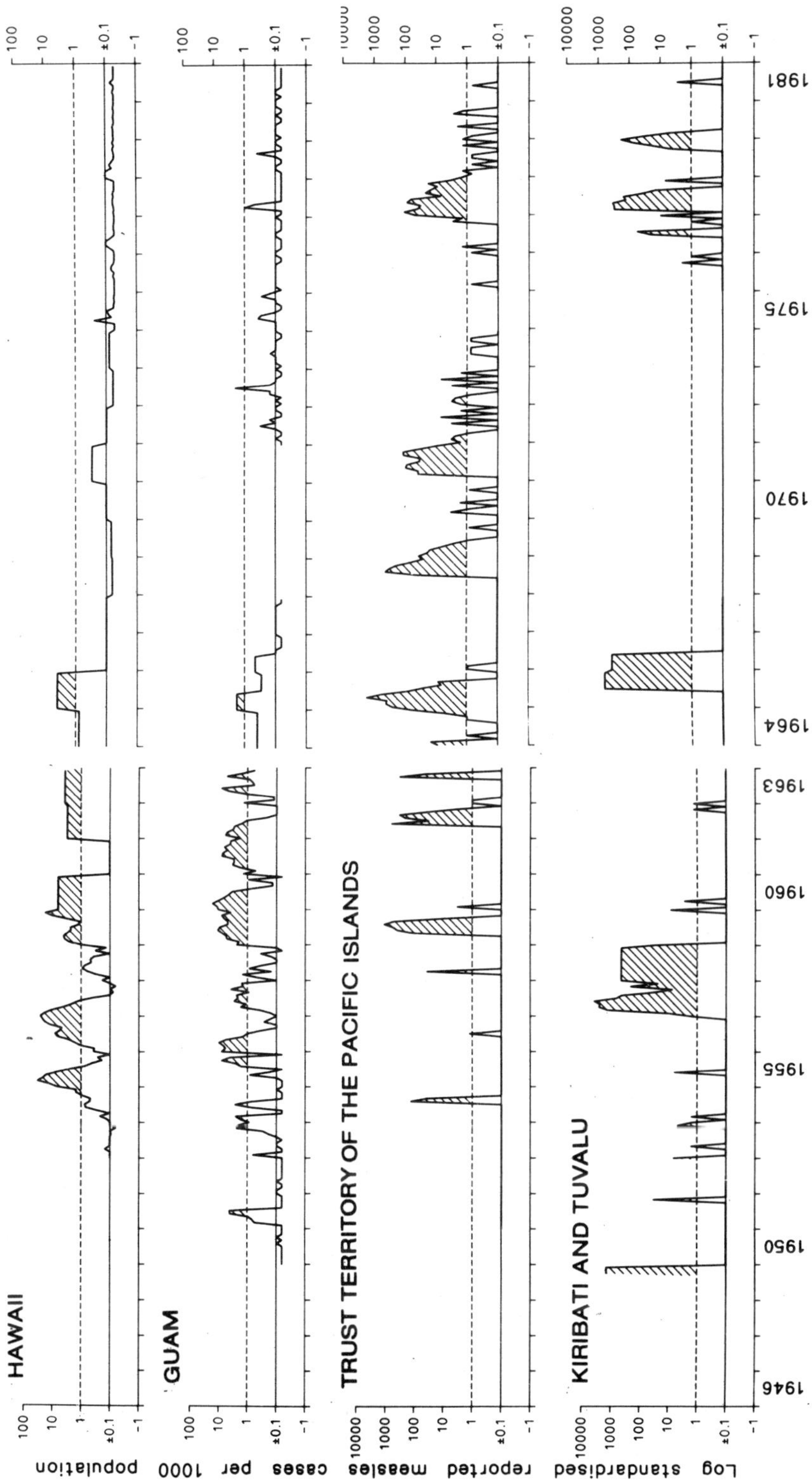

Figure 15: Monthly incidence of reported measles cases per thousand population, 1946-81, for fourteen Pacific island systems.

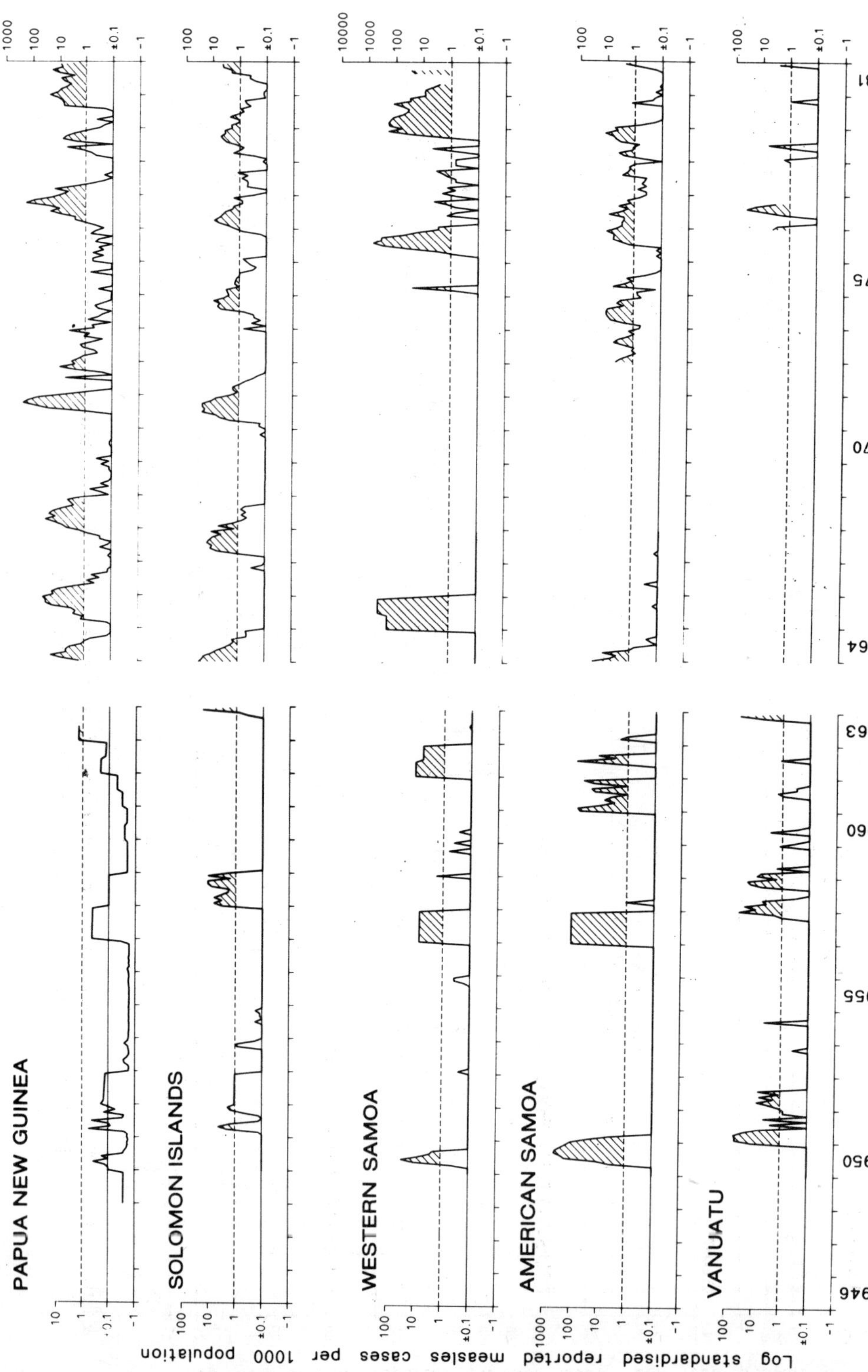

Figure 15: continued

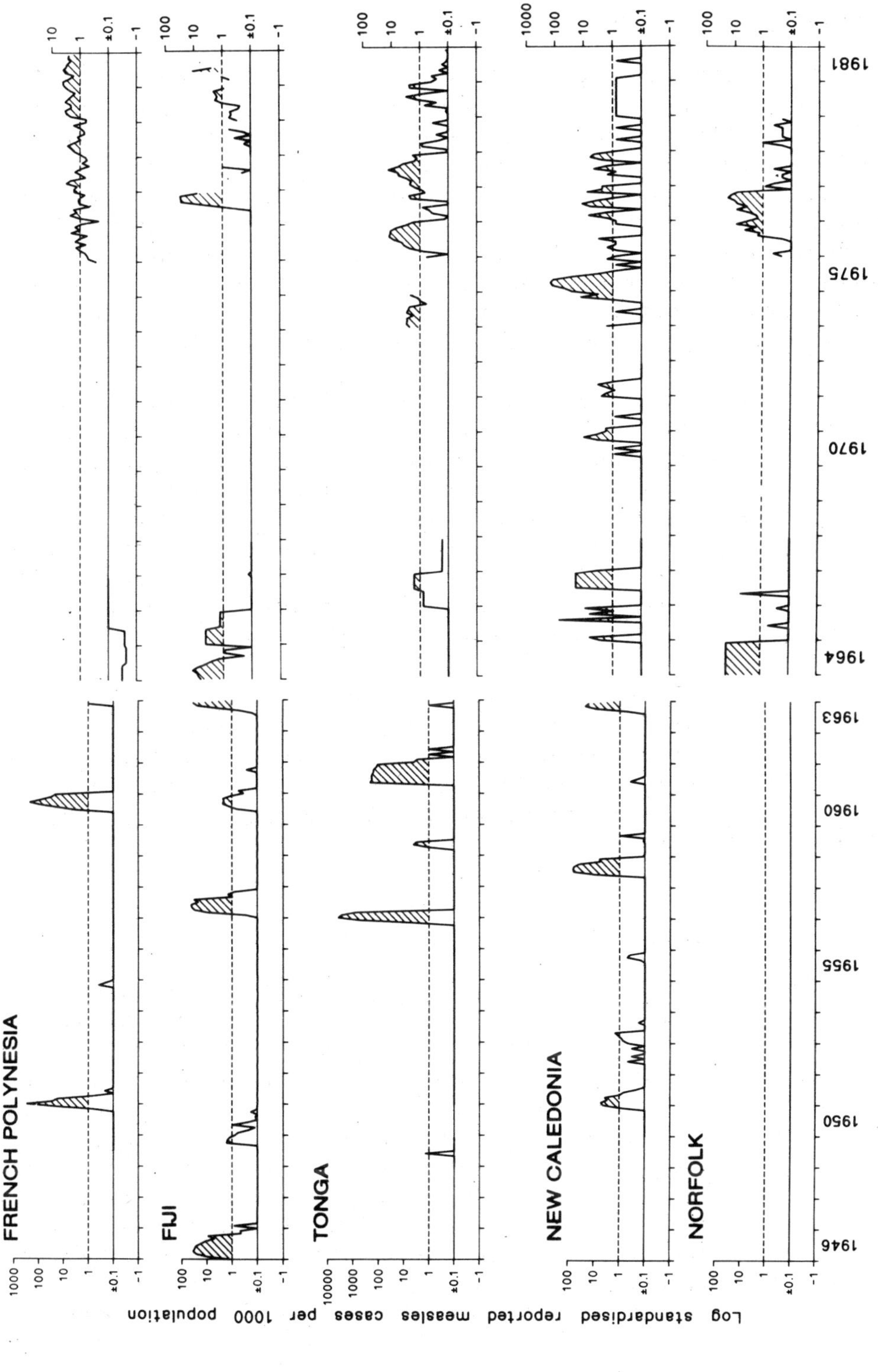

Figure 15: continued

monthly rate is plotted for the months in question. This accounts for the flat line occurring in some high-valued sections of the plots.

The series in Figure 15 have been arranged geographically by latitude from north to south, and range from the Hawaiian Islands (latitude 20°N) to Norfolk Island (27°S). Those series from countries with large populations tend to have regular outbreaks of measles and relatively low monthly variations in amplitude; the plot for Papua New Guinea is a good example. Conversely, small and isolated island groups, where an outbreak of measles may be a relatively rare event, have more dramatic contrasts and large variations in amplitude; the Tongan series illustrates the point.

The effect of the measles eradication program, launched by the United States in 1964, upon the series for Hawaii and Guam is strikingly shown in the diagram, with the elimination of anything resembling an epidemic in either series since that date. Thus, Figure 16 shows in detail the fall in measles cases in the twenty years since 1960 in the whole group and in the main Hawaiian island. For the islands as a whole, the total cases have fallen from several thousands a year in the early 1960s to less than ten a year today.

The importance of standardising data in the way undertaken here is made apparent by the Papua New Guinea series of Figure 15, where there appears to be a rising time trend in reported case rates. This is more likely to be an artefact of the improved recording system than a major change in measles incidence.

Seasonal patterns

The marked differences in amplitudes of the various series of Figure 15 is also seen when seasonal variations are considered (Figure 17). In smaller communities like Norfolk Island, with very few epidemics, the average rate for any single month is likely to reflect the accident of the month in which an introduction of measles virus occurred, rather than any recognisable seasonal cycle related to regular changes in either the physical or demographic environment. Thus, the seasonal plots in Figure 17 do not appear to show any simple or overall contrasts in levels of measles activity. Nevertheless, there are regularities that can be identified. Fiji has a clear seasonal difference between the high measles

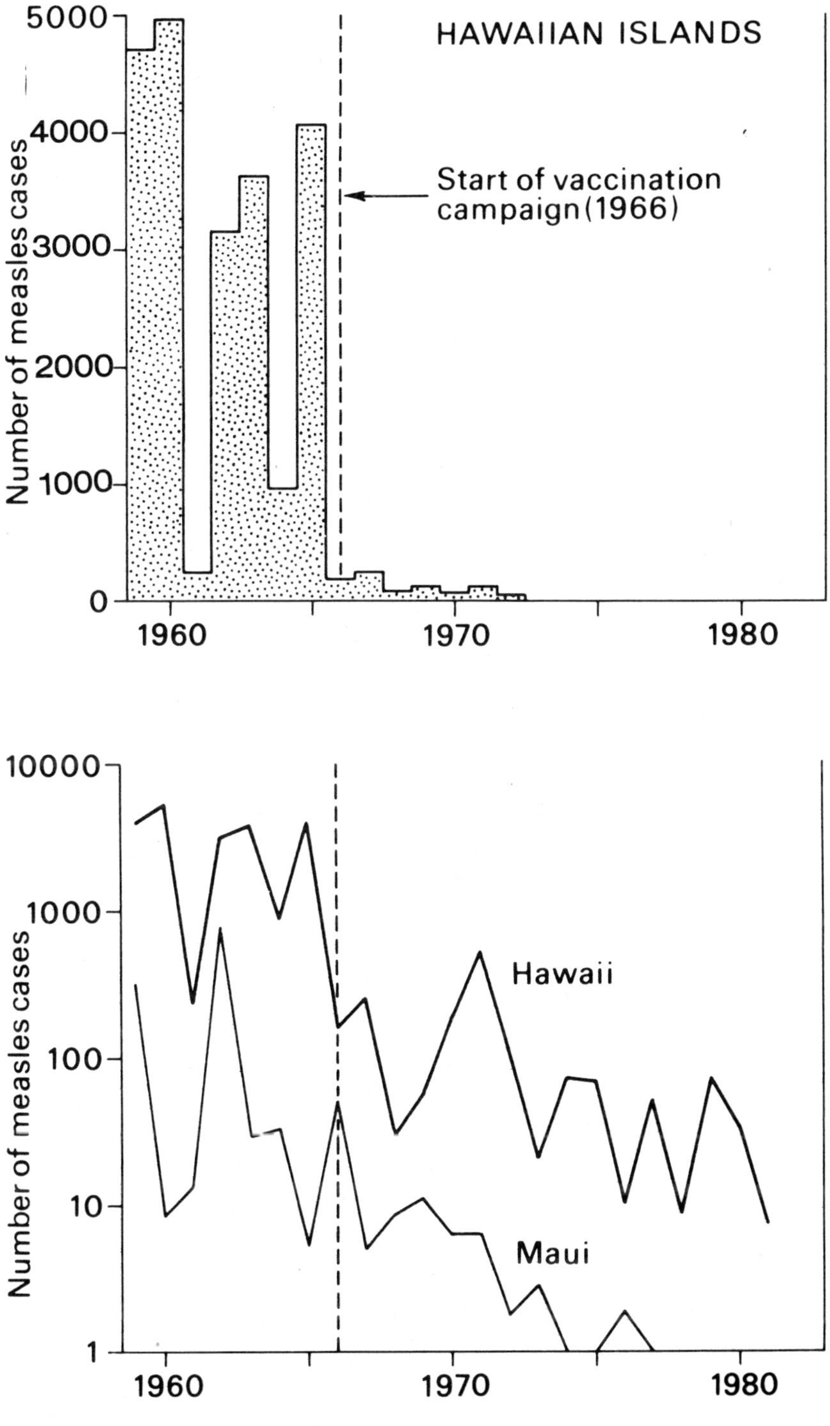

Figure 16: Measles cases in the Hawaiian Islands, 1959-81.

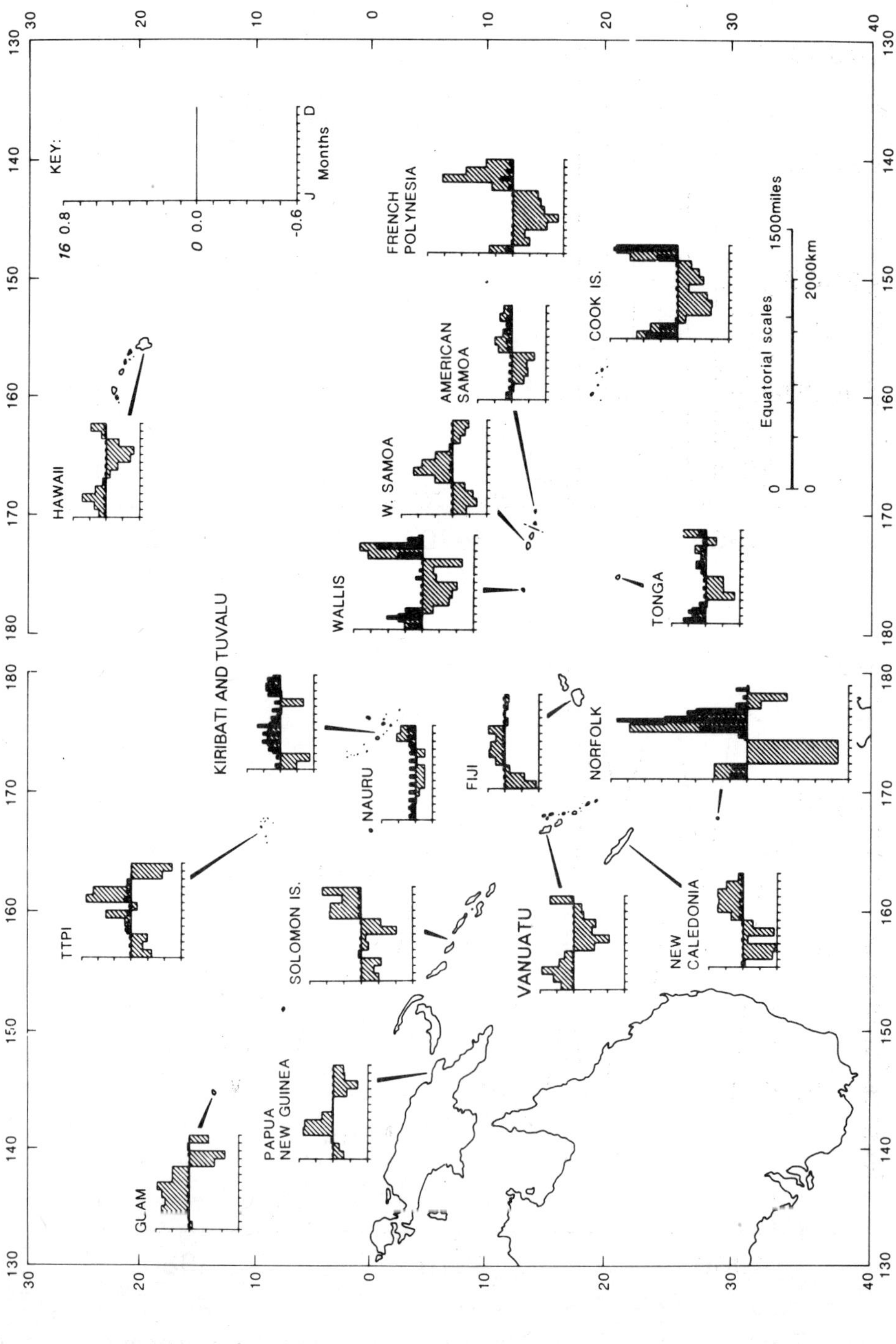

Figure 17: Average monthly incidence of reported measles cases, 1946-81

months (April through August) and the low months (September through March). This Fijian pattern is repeated in Western Samoa, the Trust Territories of the Pacific and Guam. In contrast, in Hawaii, this pattern is reversed, with the high measles months following the trend common in northern mid-latitude countries and running from November to April.

The detailed relation of measles incidence to seasonal patterns of precipitation in the Pacific (Fitzpatrick et al., 1966; Jen-Hu Chang, 1968) has yet to be fully explored. In general, we should only expect distinctive and interpretable patterns of seasonal incidence in measles to occur in communities large enough to have regular measles outbreaks.

Wave cycles: autocorrelation and partial autocorrelation functions

In order to throw light on the different wave characteristics of the measles time series for the Pacific island groups, it is useful to use autocorrelation and partial autocorrelation analysis. The method is described in Cliff and Ord (1981). In this approach, the degree of correlation in reported rates of measles per thousand population is computed for all pairs of months which are 1,2...k months apart (the lag) in the time series. The plot of autocorrelation against time lag yields a correlogram. The partial autocorrelation function gives the degree of correlation between all pairs of months in a series which are a specific lag apart, but with the effect of all other lags held constant. An illustration of the method is given in Figure 18.

The time series for Fiji since 1945 shows eleven distinctive measles peaks in a thirty-six year period. Inspection of the series indicates that it is clearly non-stationary, with the epidemic peaks decreasing in intensity and increasing in frequency over time; indeed, the Fijian series mirrors the results found in our earlier study in Iceland and represents another classic example of a regular epidemiological process at work. The autocorrelation function curve (ACF) in Figure 18 shows a secondary peak at around three to four years reflecting the average spacing of the waves. The sag in the autocorrelation curve to give negative values between six and thirty-six months confirms that the original series is not stationary; in a strictly stationary process, the ACF should be approximately zero, apart from cyclical recurrences, beyond the first few lags. Study of the partial autocorrelation curve (PACF) in Figure 18 helps to identify the nature of the process generating the pattern in the time series. Alternation of positive and negative terms, together with the damping of values of both signs over the first twelve months, suggests that the Fijian series is more appropriately modelled as a moving-average rather than an autoregressive process.

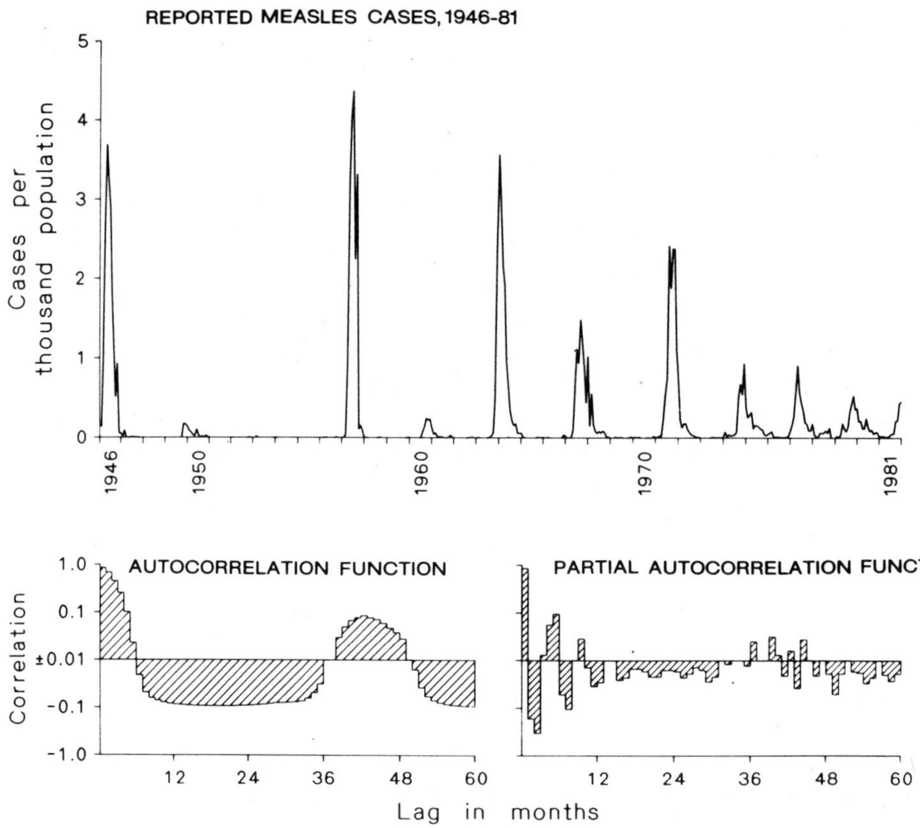

Figure 18: Reported measles cases per thousand population, monthly, for Fiji, 1946-81.

Computation of the diagnostic ACF and PACF curves for all the eighteen countries studied in the Pacific has not proved possible because of the fragmented and interrupted character of some of the measles series. Reference back to the data matrix of Figure 13 indicates that two periods or 'windows' with exceptionally full published records can be identified: a fifteen-year spell from 1953 and a five-year spell from 1976. For the earlier period, Figure 19 plots on a log scale the positive parts of the ACF which exceed 0.01. Figure 20 repeats this for the later period. Notice from the figure captions that, on both diagrams, the ACF has been computed from the longest continuous series about the relevant dates that could be constructed for any individual island; as a consequence there is considerable variation in the length of the series on which the ACF is based. In both diagrams, only the positive parts of the autocorrelation function have been plotted. Lags are shown up to a maximum of eighty-four months or the main cyclical recurrence, whichever is the shorter.

Study of the ACFs in the two diagrams shows that cyclical recurrences in epidemic outbreaks appear to occur in two-thirds of the twenty-six series computed. As we noted earlier, Fiji has a three to four-year cycle, and this shows up clearly in Figure 19. We would expect islands which are either larger or have unusually close communications with mainland reservoir areas to have shorter cycles; the two-year peaks for Guam and Hawaii fit this generalisation. But over most of the Pacific islands studied, the cycles are much longer and range from four to seven years.

Between the periods represented by the two maps, the Pacific island populations have become both larger and better connected to the outside world, and it would be tempting to see the shortening in the length of cycles between the first and second maps as reflecting these trends.

The average cycle lengths identified above are consistent with Black's findings summarised earlier in Figure 1. In Figure 21, Black's approach has been applied to the various Pacific island groups. The proportion of months with reported measles cases against population size has been plotted on log scales. With the exception of Fiji, the average values calculated from data covering the period 1950-81 have been used. For Fiji, the relationship has been estimated for four periods, namely, 1946-55; 1956-65; 1966-75; 1977-81. Comparison of Figure 21 with Figure 1 shows the same positive relationship between the two variables and the temporal

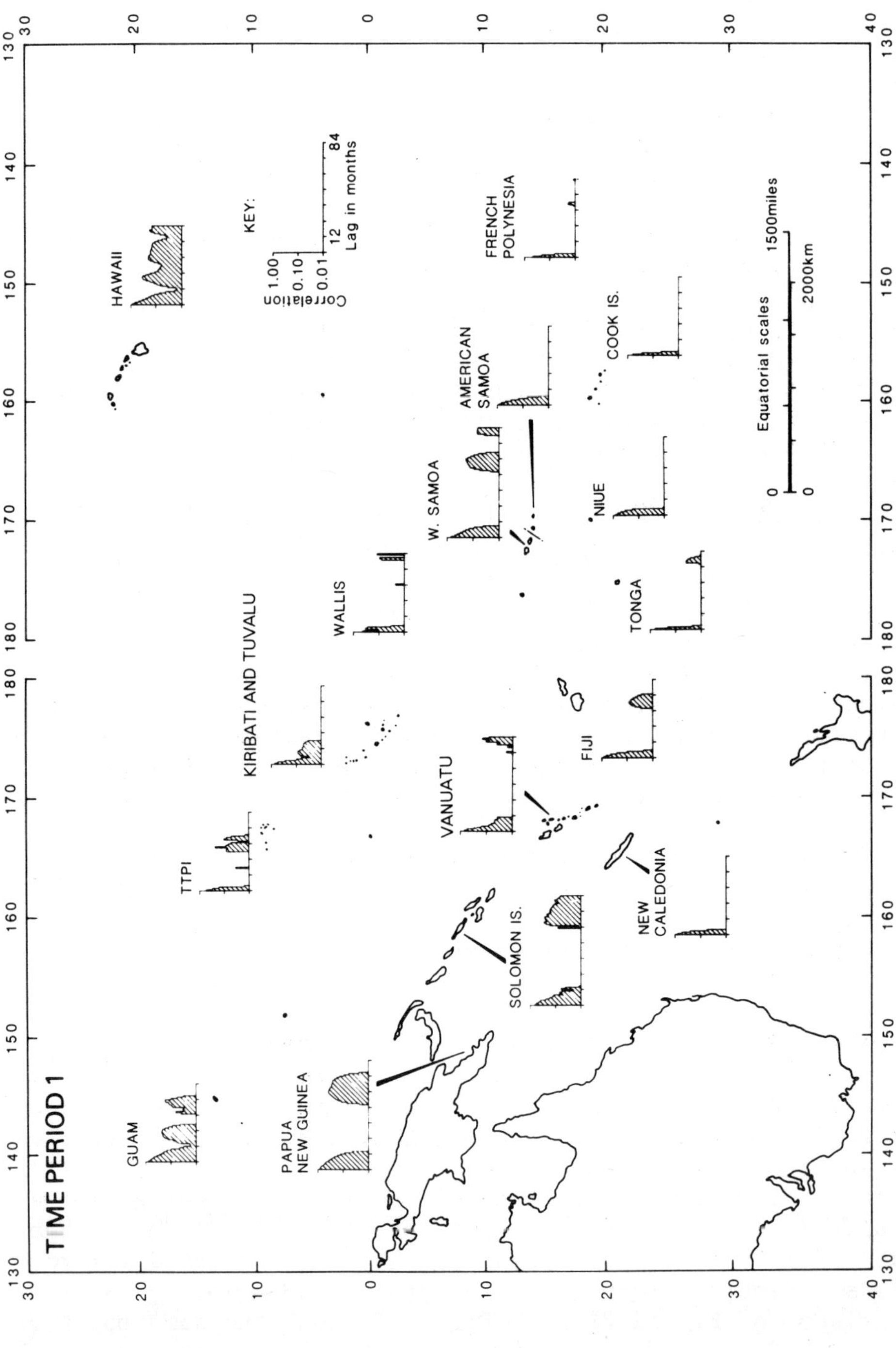

Figure 19: Plot of the positive parts of the autocorrelation functions (logarithmic scale) for sixteen Pacific islands.

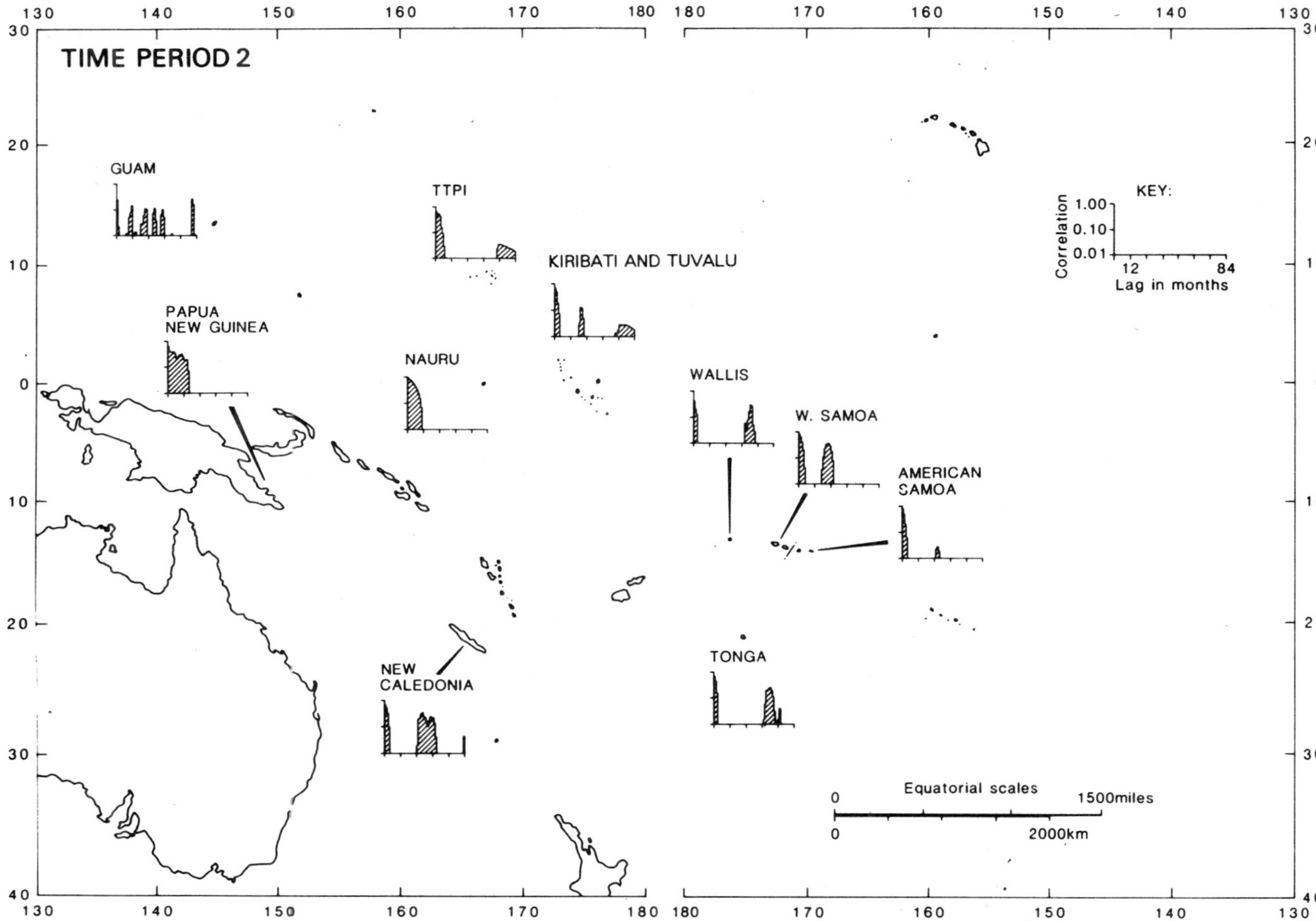

Figure 20: Plot of the positive parts of the autocorrelation functions (logarithmic scale) for ten Pacific islands.

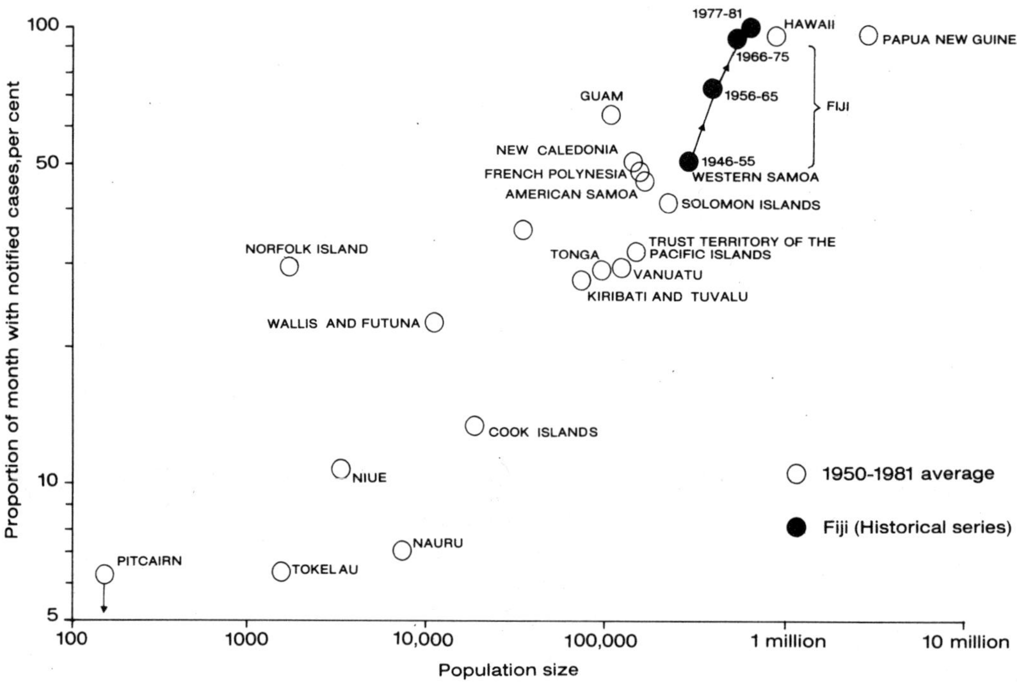

Figure 21: The relationship between proportion of months with notified measles cases and population size for twenty-one Pacific island groups, 1950-81.

migration of Fiji up the graph to its current position of measles endemicity and population of over 600,000. This mirrors the position of Hawaii in Black's original work.

Geographical integration: a qualitative approach

The relationship of Fiji to the other island groups in the Pacific can be pursued by several means. One approach is to comb the medical reports for hints of cross-infections between the island groups. Occasionally the Fijian annual reports refer to such transfers. For example, the 1946 report notes that the epidemic there has been 'spread to the British Solomon Islands Protectorate and arrived in the Gilbert and Ellice Islands colony quite independently from Johnston Island in the north'.(24) But as the volume of inter-island and external contacts grow, particularly with air travel, the contacts are ever harder to trace and very few measles index cases are identifiable. In those circumstances, we have to search for an alternative mode of analysis by plotting the pattern of infections and drawing inferences about transfer. In this sub-section, the sources are examined and two analytical channels are explored.

Evidence for other Pacific islands. As we have seen, it is not possible, as it is with Fiji, to develop a complete and comparable series for the other score of Pacific countries examined in this paper. The records in the late nineteenth and early twentieth centuries are fragmentary and incomplete and, even when available, are based on different sources. The number of recorded measles cases may be based on hospital admissions in some areas and on medical officer reports on others. Almost invariably, the reported figures are underestimates and must be treated with great caution.

With the setting up of the South Pacific Health Service in 1946, the situation improves rapidly. For under its general provision an Epidemiological Service was also inaugurated. Member states sent coded telegrams of the location of first cases and of measures taken to prevent the spread of the disease (e.g. vaccination, restriction of movement of local vessels, etc.). This was followed by weekly summaries of new cases up to the disappearance of the disease. A regular digest of the progress of outbreaks was sent from the central office in Suva to participating countries.(25)

Analysis: the 1956-58 wave. There are two main ways of exploring the links between Fiji and other island groups using these data. The first is to take a major wave which affects several island groups (including Fiji) and to trace its spread across the Pacific. The largest wave in the post-war period appears to have occurred in the late 1950s, with a sharp peak in January 1957 (Figure 15 earlier peak).

If we take the three year period around this, we can decompose it into its separate spatial components. The years 1956 to 1958 were ones of high activity in the Pacific with more than 44,000 measles cases being reported. Several groups (Tonga, Cook Islands and the Gilbert and Ellice) had their most severe epidemics for over a decade, while only French Polynesia, Pitcairn and Norfolk Island failed to report cases. In the case of Fiji itself, the period overlaps with Wave VIII, the third largest in the period since notified cases were available.

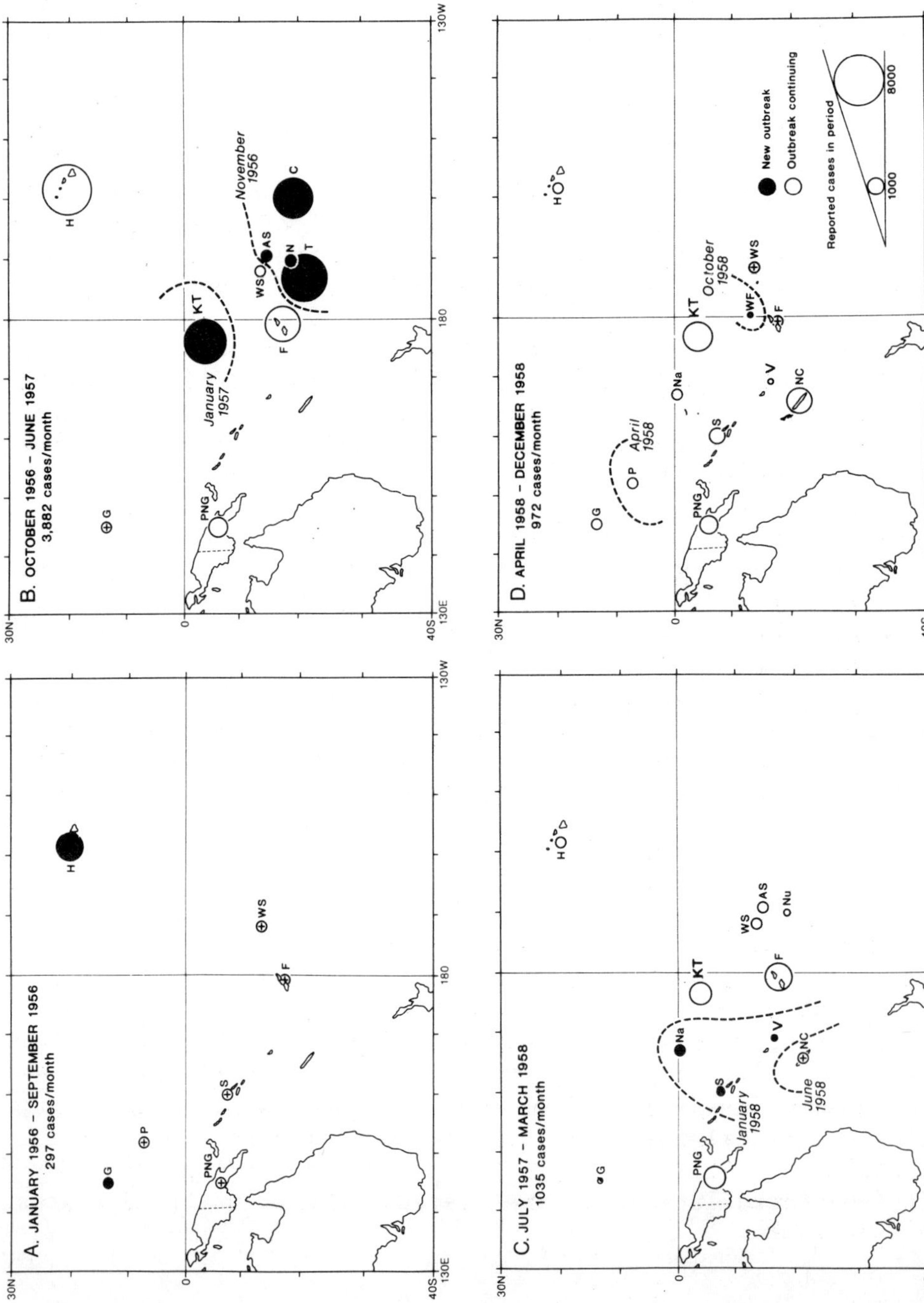

Figure 22: Measles incidence in the islands of the Pacific basin, 1956-58, for four nine-month periods.

The geographical pattern can be followed in the four maps of Figure 22. In the first nine months, activity is at a low level with Hawaii and Guam in the northern Pacific as the two main centres. Towards the end of 1956, both Fiji and Western Samoa in the central Pacific report increasing numbers of cases, while wholly new and severe epidemics begin from November 1956 towards the south-east (American Samoa, Tonga, Cook Islands and Niue) and from January 1957 towards the north-west (Kiribati and Tuvalu). In the third map, the level of activity drops by about one quarter, but new epidemics have started in the south-west quadrant. Nauru, the Solomon Islands and the New Hebrides report outbreaks from January 1958. Further south, New Caledonia reports a small outbreak in June 1958. In the fourth map, the level of activity falls only slightly, but outbreaks in the south-west quadrant continue to develop strongly while falling away in the rest of the Pacific. The only wholly new outbreak is a small one in the U.S. Pacific Island Territories in April 1958.

Given the different rates of reporting, the detailed differences in the maps in Figure 22 should be treated with caution. For example, there may well be over-reporting in the case of Kiribati and Tuvalu and under-reporting in the case of Papua New Guinea. But given the massive level of cases recorded, the general sequence is probably correct. One way of compensating for minor reporting differences is to compare the general shape and timing of the cumulative sum curves. Figure 23 plots these in logarithmic form for the three years. Islands with a continuous record of notified cases (Hawaii, Fiji, and Guam) have been separated (A) from those which exhibit a sudden burst of activity (B). This latter group shows a distinct pattern with the tracks of the south-west group (Solomons, Vanuatu, New Caledonia) lagging some six to eighteen months behind the central and south-east group (Cooks, Tonga, Kiribati and Tuvalu).

Geographical interpretation: a quantitative approach

One powerful way of measuring the association between two time series is through the use of cross-correlation functions (CCFs). The principle behind the CCF is shown in Figure 24, in which the measles records for Fiji are related to those of the Cook Islands over the 180 months from January 1953. As the lower curve shows, the correlation between the two series is $r = 0.041$ when the two series are in phase. However, the maximum correlation ($r = +0.63$) is achieved when the two

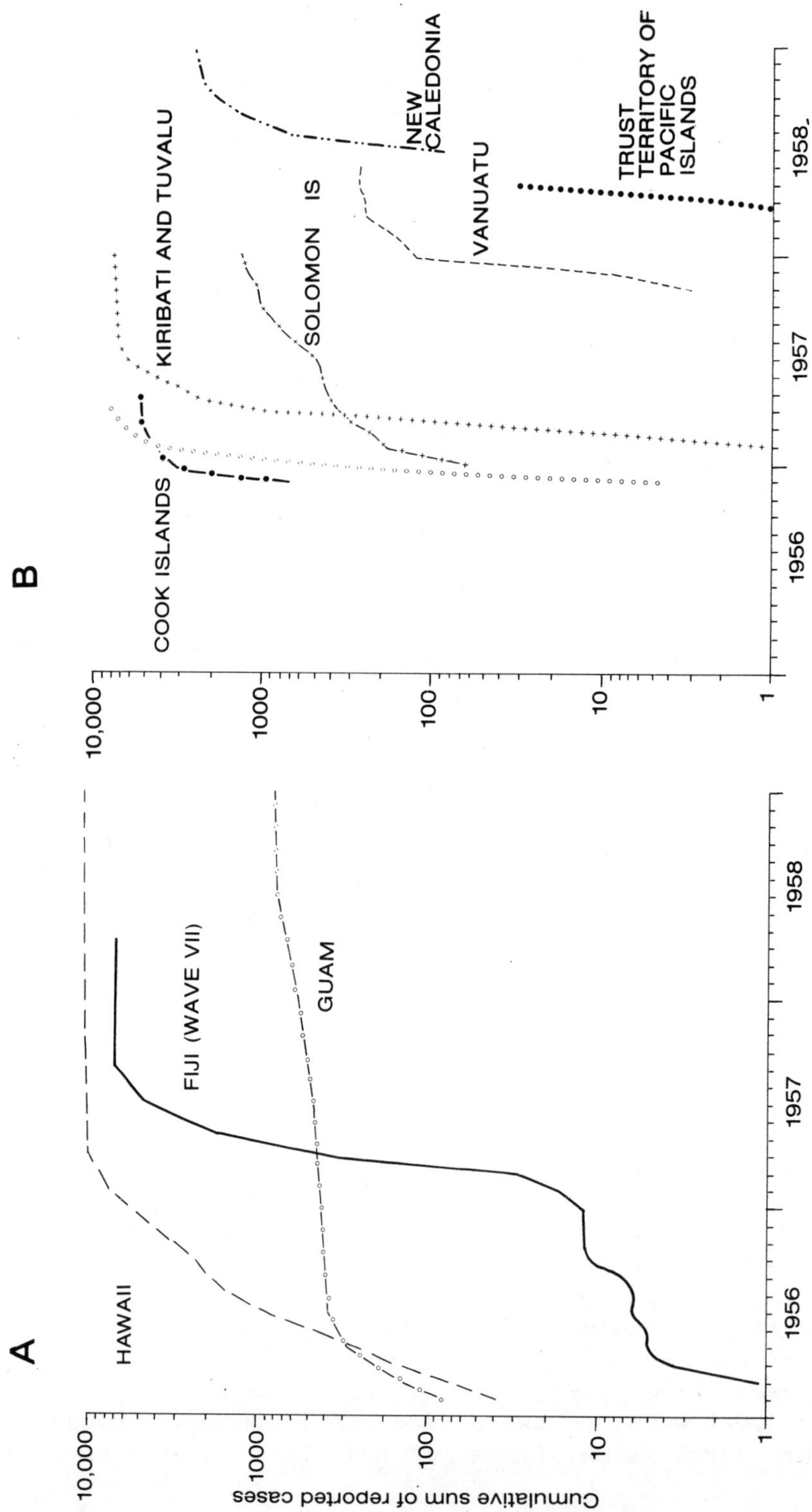

Figure 23: Diffusion curves for measles incidence in the countries of the Pacific basin between 1956 and 1958.

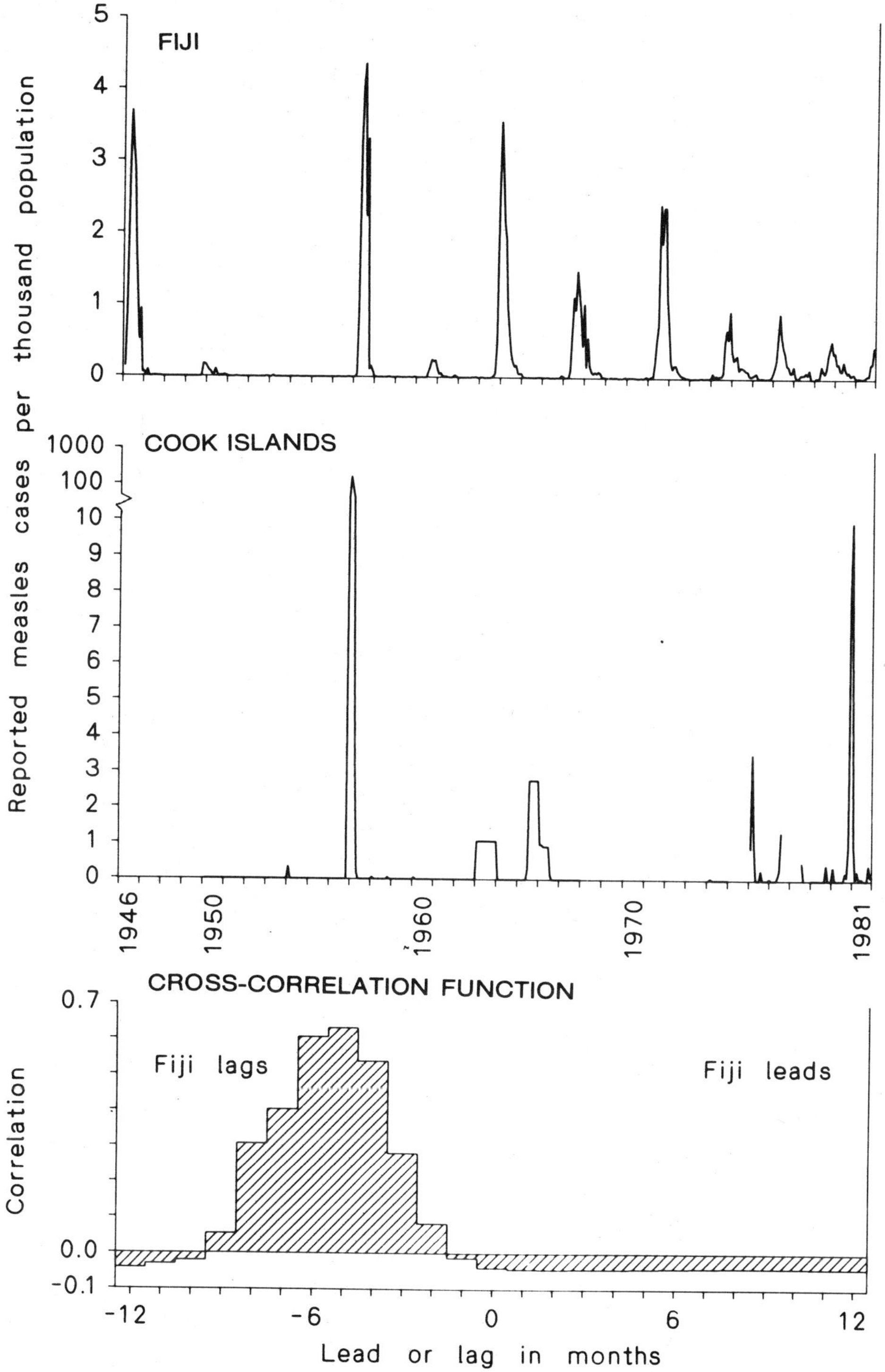

Figure 24: Reported cases of measles per thousand population, 1953-67 for Fiji and the Cook Islands.

series are out of phase by five months. This may be interpreted as Fiji 'lagging' the Cooks by five months (or equally as the Cooks 'leading' Fiji by the same interval). It is important to recognise that cross-correlation analysis measures only the coherence and phase characteristics between pairs of series. It does not imply that there is a causal link, such that changes in the leading series necessarily cause changes in the lagging series, still less (in this context) that the measles virus is transferred in the direction of such a lag. However, absence of lags, together with a high correlation, would suggest two island groups showed very similar epidemiological behaviour over time; conversely, a high lead or lag together with a low correlation would imply very dissimilar behaviour.

Thus, when we look at the pattern of leads and lags over the whole study area for the two time periods (Figures 25 and 26), the result is predictably complex. For the first time period, study of the CCFs between the major island groups suggests two geographically discrete sub-systems; each sub-system has a distinctive cross-correlation structure. The first, in the western Pacific, consists of the Solomons, Vanuatu, New Caledonia and the Trust Territories of the Pacific. Here leads and lags range up to two months. The second is the eastern Pacific and consists of Fiji, Tonga, the Cooks, the two Samoas, Kiribati and Tuvalu, with leads and lags of up to five months. Outside these two regional sub-systems, and with little statistical association with them, lie Guam, Hawaii and French Polynesia, where little correlation is likely in view of their different patterns of external linkages.

The cross-correlations in the second time period yield a different pattern (Figure 26). The vectors display a stronger east-west component, with a very large number of links focussing on French Polynesia. The places which were outside the two regional sub-systems in the first time period now appear to be more closely connected into the overall system.

These results may have important epidemiological implications. Particularly striking is the contrast between the two time periods in the overall level of cross-correlations between the pairs of time series. If all the links between the island groups are plotted as histograms (Figure 27), then some idea of the general level of

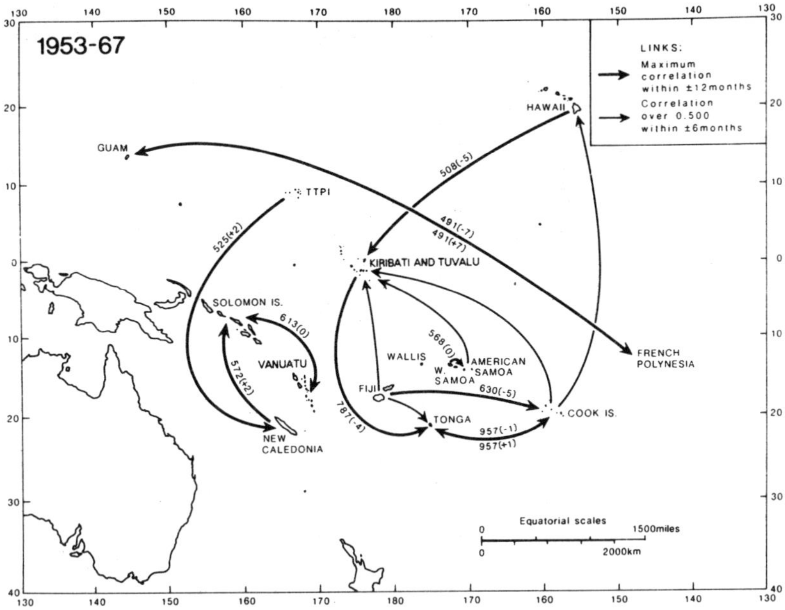

Figure 25: Spatial patterns of leads and lags between fourteen Pacific island systems based upon a cross-correlation analysis of reported measles cases per thousand population, 1953-67

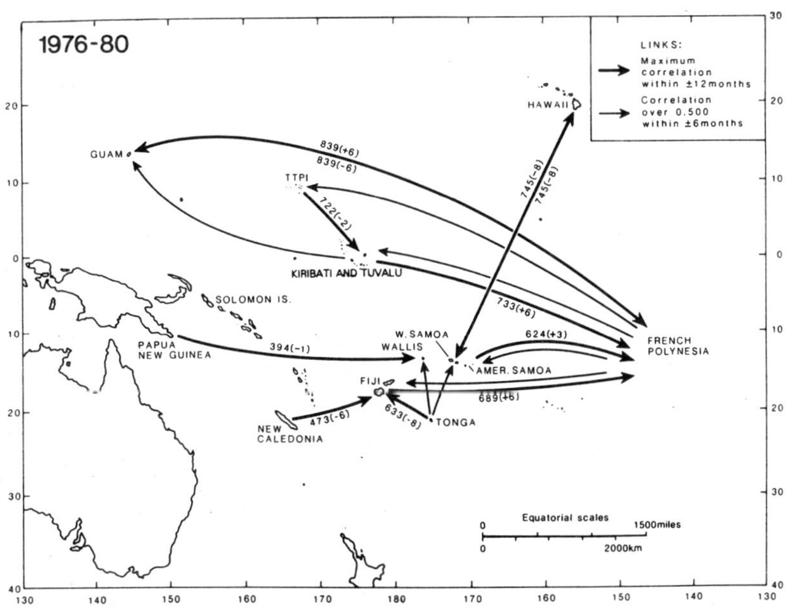

Figure 26: Spatial pattern of leads and lags between fourteen Pacific island systems based upon a cross-correlation analysis of reported measles cases per thousand population, 1976-80

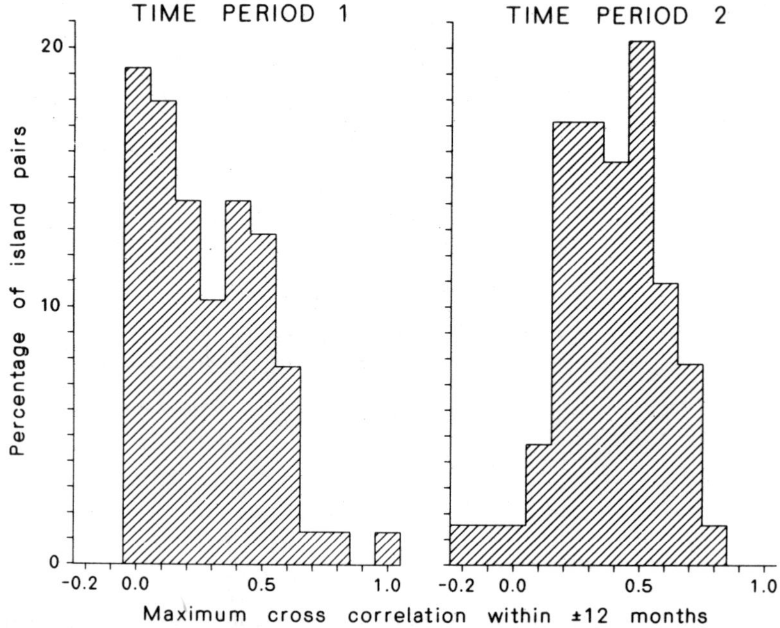

Figure 27: The percentage of island pairs in the cross-correlation analysis whose maximum cross-correlation value occurred in unit classes with -0.2, 1.0 and leads or lags of up to twelve months.

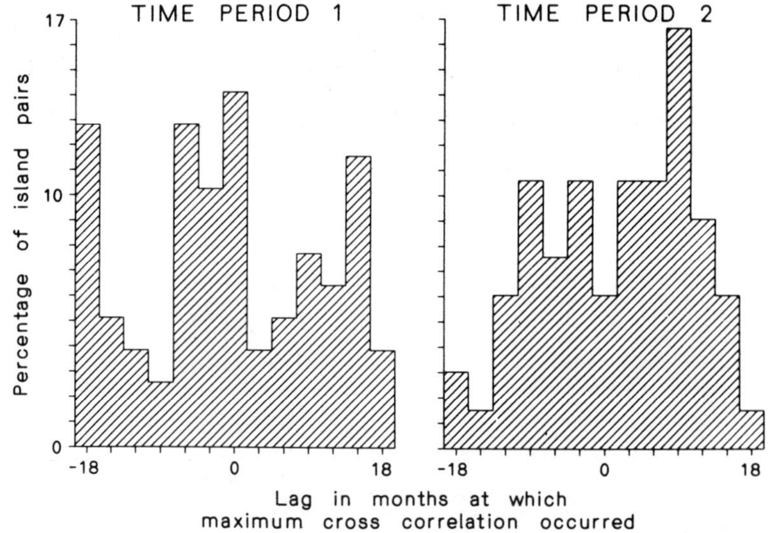

Figure 28: The percentage of island pairs in the cross-correlation analysis whose maximum cross-correlation value occurred at various lags up to eighteen months.

association can be gained. In the first period, the modal value for the maximum cross-correlation coefficient was zero; for the second period it was r = +0.6. This increase in the level of association between all time series studied is statistically significant.

The increase in coherence is also underlined by the nature of the lag structures. In Figure 28, the lag in months at which the maximum CCF value was obtained within a period of plus or minus seventeen months is plotted. In the first histogram, the proportion of links falling in the extreme classes representing leads and lags of a year or more is much greater than in the second period.

It is possible that the increasing coherence with time is due to the increased contact between islands brought about by air transport improvements. This would increase the rate of virus circulation and allow less time for large stocks of susceptible individuals to build up. Parallel arguments on the impact of transport movements on the spread of malaria in the southwest Pacific have been put forward by R.H. Black (1956).

We reiterate that the vectors shown in Figure 25 and 26 do not imply movements of the measles virus between the island groups in the direction of the vectors. As we stated earlier, CCFs merely indicate which pairs of series are similar or dissimilar in terms of their time-series properties. Any strict epidemiological interpretation would, in any case, clearly be invalidated by the absence from the analysis of major virus-reservoir areas around the Pacific margin. We would, of course, have analysed measles morbidity data for Australia and New Zealand had these data been available; in view of the absence of such data there seemed little point in including more peripheral areas such as the United States and Japan for which data series do exist.

CONCLUSIONS

The spread of measles into the island populations of the Pacific appears to have been mainly a nineteenth century phenomenon. In 1800, measles seem to have been unknown in the Pacific; by 1900 it had visited most of the main island groups at least once. The increasing volume of contacts and the decreasing travel times in this century allowed the virus to be transmitted ever more freely, particularly once new reservoir areas for the virus had been established on the Pacific margins in the southwest (Australia and New Zealand) and in western North America.

A study of epidemics in the Fijian group of islands showed that fourteen distinct measles waves have occurred since 1875. These range in character from the first, in which there was at least 28,000 and perhaps as many as 40,000 deaths, to the most recent in which no deaths from measles resulted in a population four times as large. The provenance of the waves showed Australia as a major source, with the role of Indian immigrants less important than had been previously assumed.

O.H.K. Spate has drawn attention to two histories of the Pacific, one 'oceanic' and broad in geographic scale, the other 'insular' and highly focussed (Spate, 1978:32-45). The transmission of infectious diseases shows, as Spate went on to argue, that these two themes are closely interlinked and that the events on a single island mirror the larger drama in the Pacific basin as a whole. The methods of time-series analysis enabled us to establish that epidemics on Fiji could not be regarded as independent of those on other islands in the Pacific. Indeed, the evidence of cross-correlation analysis supports the view that the various island groups have become more closely bonded together over time in terms of their epidemiological behaviour, probably as a result of modern transport developments.

If the first acts of the history of measles in the Pacific were dominated by tragedy, the present stage is one of some optimism. There is some hope that a geographical extension of the wholesale vaccination against measles currently undertaken in the United States would permit the reduction and eventual elimination of the disease in the region.

NOTES

1. Report of the Commission, op.cit., p.164.

2. Letter from Alexander H. Gordon, J.P. Nandi to his father, The Rev. John Gordon, Lisburn, Ireland, March 1875 published in The Times, London, 10 July 1875, p.6.

3. The Times, London, Wednesday June 30, 1875, p.5.

4. idem., p.5.

5. H. Silvester-Evans, Chief Medical Officer, Annual Medical Report, 1946. Fiji. Legislative Council Papers, No.6, 1947, p.4.

6. Fiji. Blue book, Levuka, 1876. Table I, p.185. 'Number, Tonnage and crews of sailing vessels entered at Ports in the Colony of Fiji from each Country in the Year 1876'.

7. idem., p.146.

8. We are grateful to Professor R.G. Ward for this suggestion.

9. 'April 8. Wellington, N.Z. Measles very prevalent here'. Fiji Times, Levuka, Wednesday April 28, 1875.

10. A.W. Campbell, District Medical Officer, Rewa. In Medical Department report, 1918. Fiji. Legislative Council Paper, No.31, 1919, p.24.

11. G.C. Strathcairn, Annual Medical Report, 1920. Fiji. Legislative Council Paper, No.43, 1921, p.5.

12. Annual Report on Indian immigration to, Indian emigration from, and indentured Indian immigrants in the Colony for the year 1911. Fiji. Legislative Council Paper, No.48, 1912, p.3.

13. Report on Indian Immigrations, etc. 1902. Fiji. Legislative Council Paper, No.20, 1903, p.3.

14. Report on Indian Immigrations, etc. 1902. Fiji. Legislative Council Paper, No.20, 1903, p.2.

15. idem., p.2.

16. V.W.T. McGusty, *Annual Medical and Health Report, 1937. Fiji. Legislative Council Paper, No.43, 1938*, p.5.

17. *Report of the Commission*, op.cit., p.31.

18. K. Gravelle, *A history of Fiji*. Suva, Fiji Times 1981, p.141.

19. A. Montague, *Annual Medical Report, 1921*. Fiji. Legislative Council Paper, No.51, 1922, p.4.

20. M.J. McCawley, District Medical Officer, Nadroga. In *Annual Medical Report 1927*. Fiji. Legislative Council Paper, No.57, 1928, p.28.

21. C.H. Gurd, *Annual Medical Report 1963*. Fiji. Legislative Council Paper, No.24, p.1, 1964.

22. C.H. Gurd, *Annual Medical Report 1967*. Fiji. Legislative Council Paper, No.37, p.13, 1968.

23. idem., p.13.

24. H. Silvester-Evans, *Annual Medical Report, 1946*. Fiji. Legislative Council Paper, No.6, 1947, p.4.

25. A full description of the reporting procedures is given in the annual *Inspector General's Report, South Pacific Health Service*. 1946-.

APPENDICES

Appendix I. Documents

(a) Letter from the Chief Medical Officer to the Colonial Secretary, Levuka, dated 7th September 1875, reporting deaths from the Windward Islands since the visit of the *Barracouta*.

(b) Letter from the Chief Medical Officer to the Colonial Secretary, Levuka, dated 8th September 1875, giving details of an interview with Mr Young from Ono, also the estimates of deaths at Ono from measles.

(c) Letter from the Office of the Stipendiary Magistrate, Lomaloma, Fiji, dated 18th November 1875, giving 'Final Return of Deaths' in the Lau district from measles.

Appendix I(a)

Levuka, Fiji 7th September, 1875

Sir,

I have the honour to forward for the information of His Excellency the Governor a copy of a letter I received yesterday:-

Tomachi, Cicia, 31st August 75

Dear Sir,

I have just received a report from the Windward islands and hasten to send you a copy for although late it may be of service to you viz. At Ono 85 deaths are reported since the visit of the "Barracouta", Lakemba 220, Namaika 40, Oniata 120, Vulaga 90, Komo 19, Kabara 89, Moce 58, Nayan 50, Vanua Vatu 4, Cicia 152, Total 842.

My informant writes me that with the exception of Ono and Vatia the measles have entirely disappeared and the general health of the Natives good. Dated August 23rd.
The Honble The Colonial Secretary

No returns from Vatoa. Some native towns are in a filthy state and we have no authority to enforce the inhabitants to cleanse them.

I remain
Dear Sir
Yours obediently
I.M. Lenox
The Health Officer
Levuka
I have the honour to be
Sir
your obedient servant

W. McGregor M.D.
C.M. Officer

Appendix I(b)

Levuka, Fiji, 8th September, 1875

Sir,

In reference to our conversation this morning on the subject of measles at Ono, I have the honour to inform you that I have an interview with the Mr. Young that left that island about a week ago.

2. He estimates the deaths at Ono from measles at 190, 120 of that number being men, and the remainder chiefly young children, with a comparatively small number of women. The epidemic is over and the general health appears to be pretty much the same as other Windward islands. He does not believe there was a single case of measles there when he left.

3. He states that the chief is alive, but that Levi the teacher is dead.

4. Mr. Young does not think it necessary to send down a medical officer as there is nothing special now requiring his presence, and as the epidemic has run itself out I agree with his opinion. Should The Governor, however, deem it advisable to send down a medical officer, Mr. Young will be going thither in a few days.

I have the honour to be,

Sir

Your obedient servant

W.McGregor M.D. C.M. Officer

Appendix I(c)

Office Stipendiary Magistrate
Lomaloma
18 November 1875

Sir,

I have the honour herewith to forward to you the Census of Lau 1875 which I have at last been enabled to compile.

also

Final Return of Deaths consequent on Measles.
Possibly this may be somewhat in excess of the number actually attributable to the said epidemic for the natives laid all deaths during the time it prevailed to that cause.
I have not hitherto mentioned I believe that a Mr. Lomberg of Cicia has been most energetic during the time of sickness in attending to the neighbouring natives and that doubtless to his care the people on the next town to where is is located owe their comparative small loss - I consider it but right to place this on record.

I have the honour to be
Sir
Your obedient servant
Horace G.C. Emberson

To the Honble the
Colonial Secretary
Levuka

REFERENCES

Part 1: Archival and Statistical Sources

A. Manuscript sources: National Archives, Suva.

Fiji. Correspondence. Inward letter to the Colonial Secretary, Fiji, 1875-76.

Fiji. Methodist Missionary Society Archives.

B. Printed sources

(1) Fiji

Fiji. Blue Books. 1890+.

Fiji. Legislative Council. Journal and Papers (1910+). Annual Medical Report of the Chief Medical Officer.

Fiji. Legislative Council. Journal and Papers. Annual Reports on Indian Immigration, etc.

Fiji. Report of the Commission appointed to inquire into the decrease of the native population. 1896.

Fiji Argus, Levuka. 1875.

Fiji Times, Levuka. 1875.

(2) Others

World Health Organization, Geneva. Epidemiological and Vital Statistics Reports.

World Health Organization, Geneva. World Health Statitics Annual.

League of Nations, Geneva. Health Section. Epidemiological Report.

League of Nations, Geneva. Health Section. Quarterly Bulletin.

South Pacific Commission. South Pacific Health Service. Inspector Generals' Report, 1946+.

South Pacific Commission. Annual Epidemiological Report, 1960+.

Centers for Disease Control, Atlanta. United States Department of Health. Morbidity and Mortality Weekly Report.

Great Britain: Parliamentary Papers. London: H.M.S.O.

The Times, London. 1876.

Sydney Gazette, Sydney. 1826+.

Part 2: Printed Papers and Books

Adels, B.R. et al., 1963, 'Survey of measles patterns in New Guinea, Micronesia and Australia, with a report on new virgin soil epidemics and the demonstration of susceptible primitive population by serology', _American Journal of Hygiene_, 77, 317-43.

Ambrosch, F., Wiedermann, G and Harasek, G., 1978, 'Costs and benefits of measles vaccination', _Fortschritte der-Medizin_, 96, 409-14.

Bailey, N.T.J., 1975, _The Mathematical Theory of Infectious Diseases_ (London: Griffin).

Bailey, N.J.T., 1981, 'Spatial models in the epidemiology of infectious diseases', _Lecture Notes in Biomathematics_, 38, 233-61.

Bartlett, M.S., 1957, 'Measles periodicity and community size', _Journal of the Royal Statistical Society, Series A_, 12, 49-70.

Black, F.L., 1966, 'Measles periodicity in insular populations: critical community size and its evolutionary implications', _Journal of Theoretical Biology_, 11, 207-11.

Black, F.L., 1976, 'Measles', in Alfred S. Evans (ed.), _Viral Infections of Humans, Epidemiology and Control_ (New York: Plenum Medical Book Company), 297-316.

Black, F.L., Pinheiro, F. de P., Hierholzer, W.J. and Lee, R.V., 1977, 'Epidemiology of infectious disease: the example of measles', in *Health and Disease in Tribal Societies* (Amsterdam: Ciba Foundation Symposium, New Series, Elsevier), 49, 115-35.

Black, F.L. and Rosen, L., 1962, 'Patterns of measles antibodies in residents of Tahiti and their stability in the absence of re-exposure', *Journal of Immunology*, 88, 725-31.

Black, R.H., 1956, 'The epidemiology of malaria in the southwest Pacific: changes associated with increasing European contact', *Oceania*, 27, 136-42.

Brookfield, H.C. with Hart, D., 1971, *Melanesia: a Geographical Interpretation of an Island World* (London: Methuen).

Brown, P., Bashight, M. and Gajdusek, D.C., 1965, 'Response to live attenuated measles vaccine in susceptible island populations of Micronesia', *American Journal of Epidemiology*, 82, 115-22.

Brown, P., Gajdusek, D.C. and Tsai, T., 1969, 'Persistence of measles antibody in the absence of circulating natural virus five years after immunization of an isolated virgin population with Edmonston B vaccine', *American Journal of Epidemiology*, 90, 514-18.

Christensen, P.E., Schmidt, H., Bang, H.O., Andersen, V., Jordal, B. and Jensen, O., 1953, 'An epidemic of measles in southern Greenland, 1951: measles in virgin soil', *Acta Medica Scandinavica*, 144, 450-54.

Cliff, A.D. and Haggett, P., 1984, 'Island epidemics', *Scientific American*, 250, 110-17.

Cliff, A.D., Haggett, P., Ord, J.K. and Versey, R., 1981, *Spatial Diffusion: an Historical Geography of Epidemics in an Island Community* (Cambridge: Cambridge University Press).

Cliff, A.D., Haggett, P. and Graham, R., 1983, 'Reconstruction of diffusion processes at local scales: the 1846, 1882 and 1904 measles epidemics in northwest Iceland', *Journal of Historical Geography*, 9, 347-68.

Cliff, A.D. and Ord, J.K., 1981, *Spatial Processes* (London:

Pion).

Corney, B.G., 1883-4, 'The behaviour of certain epidemic diseases in natives of Polynesia with special reference to Fiji', Epidemiological Society of London, Transactions. New Series, 3, 76-94.

Cumpston, J.H.L., 1927, The History of Diptheria, Scarlet Fever, Measles and Whooping Cough in Australia (Canberra: Commonwealth of Australia, Department of Health, Service Publication No. 37).

Fitzpatrick, E.A., Hart, D. and Brookfield, H.C., 1966, 'Rainfall seasonality in the tropical southwest Pacific', Erdkunde, 20, 181-94.

Gillion, K.L., 1962, Fiji's Indian Migrants: a History to the End of Indenture in 1920 (Melbourne: Oxford University Press).

Gould, K.L., Hermann, K.L., and Witte, J.J., 1971, 'The epidemiology of measles in the US Trust Territory of the Pacific Islands', American Journal of Public Health, 61, 1602-13.

Hinman, A.R., Bart, K.J., Orenstein, W.A., Kirby, C.D. and Bloch, A.B., 1982a, History of Measles Control Efforts. Paper presented at the Conference 'Conquest of agents that endanger the brain', Baltimore, Maryland, October 28-29, 1982.

Hinman, A.R., Amler, R.M., Bloch, A.B., Orenstein, W.A., Bart, K.J. and Turner, P.M., 1982b, Imported Measles in the United States (Atlanta: Centers for Disease Control, Immunization Division).

Hirsch, A., 1883, Handbook of Geographical and Historical Pathology (three volumes) [Translated from the second German edition by Charles Creighton] (London: The New Sydenham Society).

Jen-hu Chang, 1968, 'Rainfall in the tropical southwest Pacific', Geographical Review, 58, 142-4.

Joyce, R.B., 1971, Sir William McGregor (Melbourne: Oxford University Press).

Juptner, H. and Quinnell, E.M.A., 1965, 'Epidemiological observations during measles epidemic in the Trobriand Island, Papua', Medical Journal of Australia, 1, 538-40.

Kissling, C., 1980, International Civil Aviation in the South Pacific: A Perspective (Canberra: Australian National University, Development Studies Centre, Occasional Paper No. 19).

Lancaster, H.O., 1964, 1973, 'A bibliography of vital statistics in Australia and New Zealand', Australian Journal of Statistics, 6, 33-9; 15, 1-26.

McArthur, N., 1967, Island Populations of the Pacific (Canberra: Australian National University Press).

Maude, H.E., 1968, Of Islands and Men: Studies in Pacific History (Melbourne: Oxford University Press).

Navarunisaravi, N.B., 1970, Medical statistics in Fiji and epidemiolgy of the South Pacific (Suva: Medical Statistics Department of the Fiji Medical Department).

Norman-Taylor, W., 1963-78, Annotated bibliography of medical research in the South Pacific. Parts 1-6, South pacific Commission, Noumea, New Caledonia, Technical Papers, No. 142 (Parts 1-6).

Panum, P.L., 1940, Measles in the Faeroe Islands [Translation of Virchows Archiv Pathologie und Medizin, Vol.1, 1847] (Delta Omega Society: American Public Health Association), 492-512.

Peart, A.F.W. and Nagler, F.P., 1954, 'Measles in the Canadian Arctic, 1952', Canadian Journal of Public Health, 45, 146-56.

Rivers, W.H.R. (ed.) 1922, Essays on the Depopulation of Melanesia (Cambridge: Cambridge University Press).

Selby, P. (ed.) 1981, Influenza Epidemics: Modelling Prospects for Prediction and Control (Geneva: Sandoz Institute).

Spate, O.H.K., 1978, 'The Pacific as artefact', in N. Gunson (ed.), Pacific: Essays in Honour of H.E. Maude (Melbourne: Oxford University Press), 32-45.

Squire, W., 1882, 'On measles in Fiji', *Transactions of the Epidemiological Society of London* (Sessions 1875-76 to 1880-81), 4, 72-4.

Taylor, M. and Kissling, C., 1983, 'Resource dependence, power networks and the airline system of the South Pacific', *Regional Studies*, 17, 237-50.

Thomson, B.H., 1894, *The Diversions of a Prime Minister* (London: Blackwood and Sons).

Thornley, A.W., 1971, Methodist Missionary Society of Australia, Fiji District. Inventory of documents transferred by the Fiji Methodist Church in October-November 1964. Typescript. (Suva: National Archives of Fiji).

Tippett, A.R., 1953, 'Shifting foci of Methodist witness in Fiji, 1835-1900', in A.R. Tippett, *Historical Writings, 1947-1967* (Canberra: St Mark's Library), 1-58.

Tippett, A.R., 1974, 'The ethnopsychology of depopulation in the Pacific with special reference to Fiji', Manuscript (Canberra: St Mark's Library), 70 pp.

Walker, A.S., 1957, *The Island Campaigns* [Australia in the War of 1939-45, Series 5, Medical. Vol.3] (Canberra: Australian War Memorial).

Ward, R.G., 1965, *Land Use and Population in Fiji: a Geographical Study* (London: Department of Technical Cooperation, Overseas Research Publications, No. 9, HMSO).

Ward, R.G. and Dodge, E.S., 1967, *American Activities in the Central Pacific, 1790-1870: a History, Geography, and Ethnography Pertaining to American Involvement and Americans in the Pacific Taken from Contemporary Newspapers, etc* (Ridgewood, N.J.: Gregg Press), 5 vols.

Willis, M.F. and Warburton, M.F., 1974, 'Measles susceptibility in two Pacific atoll populations: epidemiological factors response to live attenuated measles virus', *Medical Journal of Australia*, 1, 789-93.

Winslow, J.M. (ed.) 1977, *The Melanesian Environment* (Canberra: Australian National University Press).

Wolfe, R.J., 1982, 'Alaska's great sickness, 1900: an epidemic of measles and influenza in a virgin soil population', _Proceedings of the American Philosophical Society_, 126, 91-121.

HG/1 (1969) **The People of Vila**
H.C. Brookfield and Paula Brown Glick
(out of print)

HG/2 (1969) **Manufacturing in Melbourne**
P.J. Rimmer (out of print)

HG/3 (1969) **Retailing in Melbourne**
R.J. Johnston and P.J. Rimmer (out of print)

HG/4 (1970) **Freight Forwarding in Australia**
P.J. Rimmer

HG/5 (1971) **Government Influence and the Location of Economic Activity**
G.J.R. Linge and P.J. Rimmer (eds)

HG/6 (1971) **Transport in Thailand and The Railway Decision**
P.J. Rimmer

HG/7 (1972) **Systems Theory: A Framework for Human Geographical Enquiry**
D.J. Walmsley

HG/8 (1973) **Studies of Contemporary Thailand**
R. Ho and E.C. Chapman (eds)(out of print)

HG/9 (1973) **New Hebridean Mobility: A Study of Circular Migration**
R.D. Bedford (out of print)

HG/10 (1976) **The New South Wales Wheat Frontier 1851 to 1911**
M.E. Robinson

HG/11 (1976) **Restructuring Employment Opportunities in Australia**
G.J.R. Linge (ed.)

HG/12 (1978) **Food, Shelter and Transport in Southeast Asia and the Pacific**
P.J. Rimmer, D.W. Drakakis-Smith and T.G. McGee (eds)

HG/13 (1979) **Corporations in Recession: The Australian Agricultural Machinery Industry**
D.A. Wadley

HG/14 (1980) **An Introduction to Marxist Theories of Underdevelopment**
Richard Peet (ed.)

HG/15 (1981) **Structural Change in Australia: Some Spatial and Organisational Responses**
G.J.R. Linge and J. McKay (eds)

HG/16 (1984) **Uneven Development and the Geographical Transfer of Value**
D.K. Forbes and P.J. Rimmer (eds)

HG/17 (1985) **Land, Cane and Coconuts: Papers on the Rural Economy of Fiji**
H.C. Brookfield, F. Ellis and R.G. Ward

HG/18 (1985) **The Spread of Measles in Fiji and the Pacific: Spatial Components in the Transmission of Epidemic Waves through Island Communities**
Andrew D. Cliff and Peter Haggett